LIVING THERAPY SERIES

Counselling Young Binge Drinkers

Person-Centred Dialogues

Richard Bryant-Jefferies

T0144689

Radcliffe Publishing

Oxford • Seattle

Radcliffe Publishing Ltd
18 Marcham Road
Abingdon
Oxon OX14 1AA
United Kingdom

www.radcliffe-oxford.com
Electronic catalogue and worldwide online ordering facility.

_____

British Library Cataloguing in Publication Data

A catalogue record for this book is available from the British Library.

ISBN-10 1 84619 059 2
ISBN-13 978 1 84619 059 9

Typeset by Aarontype Ltd, Easton, Bristol
Printed and bound by TJ International Ltd, Padstow, Cornwall

Contents

Foreword

The world as we know it is changing. Increasingly, we are being challenged to give up our idealistic notions of what it means to be a young person in our society and what constitutes 'normal' difficulties in adolescents and young adults. Not too long ago, in comparison to adulthood, youth was considered to be an idyllic and carefree time of life that was filled with the exploration of a world with promise. While we now recognize that this perspective is inconsistent with reality, the remnants of this view of youth lingers. Too often, the emotional distress of young people is minimized, dismissed or ignored. Many young people who struggle find themselves marginalized because of a widely held perception that the life struggles and emotional issues of youth are trivial and without basis. 'To be young is to have the time of your life!'

Those of us who have embraced the opportunity to work with adolescents and young adults as mental health professionals know all too well the depth and gravity of their emotional distress and their realities that have contributed to it. Emotional distress can be made manifest into a whole gamut of self-harming behaviors. Binge drinking is one example of a self-harming behavior that has a profound effect on the young person, on relationships with family and friends, and on the ability to effectively deal with difficult life circumstances.

Regrettably, as clinicians, we recognize that severe distress left unaddressed in adolescents and young adults has the potential to weaken the foundation required to build a healthy life as a contributing member of society. Because young people are often already marginalized, they can be left to struggle with their demons without the benefit of social support from society at large and with few services that they feel comfortable accessing.

The person-centered approach to providing therapy offers a broad lens through which to conceptualize binge drinking patterns of behavior and to design interventions that are aimed at adolescents and young adults with drinking problems. In this latest volume, Richard Bryant-Jefferies takes a close look at binge drinking as a manifestation of underlying issues causing distress in young people and demonstrates the impact of using a therapeutic approach that is founded on valuing the client's perception of reality. He presents a compelling case for using person-centered therapy with this often difficult-to-reach population. In addition to presenting a strong rationale for the appropriateness of using this approach with young binge drinkers who are reluctant to engage in therapy, he provides the reader with three important, distinct, yet interrelated perspectives of the therapeutic process: counsellor, client, and supervisor.

By providing us with insight into the internal perspective of each participant in the therapeutic encounter, Richard Bryant-Jefferies is able to shed light on the complexity of the issues that underlie persistent and destructive self-harming behaviors. The book is written to appeal to a spectrum of audiences including supervisors, practitioners, students and laypersons.

This presentation moves beyond the traditional academic approach that limits the transfer of knowledge to a restricted audience. For a parent or friend trying to understand binge drinking in a young person, this book can be a valuable resource. The book is written in such a manner that an interested person, regardless of their knowledge about binge drinking, is able to expand their understanding of the complexity of issues that may, on the surface, seem somewhat simplistic. This approach brings together theory and practice that is relevant to the practitioner and the layman alike.

In this book, the person-centered therapeutic orientation is applied to two specific cases of young people who are struggling with binge drinking behaviors. The presentation of dialogue and internal emotional experience of both the clients and counsellors helps the reader to understand the multiple layers of processing that are required as part of an emotionally corrective therapeutic experience. As a client, practitioner, or concerned family member, this book can help to pave the way to a better understanding of the underlying causes of disturbing behaviors associated with binge drinking in adolescents and young adults. It can also provide a ray of hope that the possibility for change is ever present in respectful, authentic and empathic therapeutic relationships.

Robin D Everall, PhD
Associate Professor of Counselling Psychology
University of Alberta
Edmonton, Alberta, Canada
December 2005

Foreword

There is still so much to learn about how to go about helping people through psychotherapy and counselling. This is not to say, of course, that a great deal has not already been written about all kinds of approaches or that a growing body of evidence has not accumulated about clinical effectiveness. We do know more than we did only a few years ago but it's probably fair to say that we still lack the opportunity to find out what really goes on in the consulting rooms around the country. Too often in case presentations, the emphasis is on the client's disturbance and with due reference to theory. Less attention is paid to the emotional texture of what it is that is happening between the participants involved. What is it that goes through the heads of psychotherapists and counsellors as they practise and what is on the minds of those in receipt of such practice? What is the experience on either side of the table as it were and what is developing beyond the realms of established technique and strategy?

This book does very well in its attempt to answer these questions. In the way it has been written, it opens a window to the reader to see and feel the intricacies of individual psychotherapy and counselling. Richard Bryant-Jefferies achieves this through the device of the fictional dialogue. Through his imagination, drawn from his own clinical experience, he creates stories of imaginary young people as they go through the counselling experience. The stories are well written and the portrayals are quite vivid. The description of the process is fascinating – capturing as it does so much of the uncertainties and the doubts as well as the breakthroughs, the moments of connection and illumination that make the whole experience so worthwhile.

With the use of the fictional dialogue, it is possible for the author to break free from the constraints set by the dictates of confidentiality. Not only can the reader learn about the inner feelings and thoughts of the client, but also of the counsellor's questions and self-criticisms as they in turn affect the course of counselling. The process is further elaborated through imaginary dialogues between the counsellors and their supervisors. Some people may question the validity of this device – of the very authenticity that is so singularly sought in the counselling it describes. It is, of course, well worth remembering that all case studies, no matter how well based on actual events, are fictional in the sense that so much is edited and selected. Ultimately, the reader has to trust the integrity of the author, that he is holding as faithfully as he can the essence of the cases he has in his mind.

There are so many ways in which readers can engage with this book – through absorbing themselves in the dialogues, through taking notes of the various general comments on theory and practice that the author inserts from time to time into the text and through considering various interesting points for discussion that he poses at the end of every chapter – not least the question 'Would you have taken a different approach?' In this respect, this book can be of value to any student of psychotherapy and counselling, whatever approach is being followed.

At the heart of the book are the principles and practice of the person-centred approach. In following the course of the fictional narrative, the author conjures up so much of what is the essence of the approach. The importance of the therapeutic relationship, the core conditions that sustain it, the respect for the autonomy of the individual, the faith in the actualising tendency of the client and the trust in the therapeutic process – all are fundamental and central themes in the book.

> From this theoretical perspective we can argue that the person-centred counsellor's role is essentially facilitative. Creating the therapeutic climate of empathic understanding, unconditional positive regard and authenticity creates a relational climate which encourages the client to move into a more fluid state with more openness to their own experience and discovery of a capacity towards a fuller actualising of their potential. (p. 37)

There is unquestionably a passion in this writing – and also a very firm sense of discipline.To work towards creating and ensuring the core conditions – empathy, congruence, unconditional positive regard, warm acceptance, staying with the present – is by no means an easy accomplishment and this comes through very clearly in the book. Quite stern prohibitions are laid on the counsellor – not to intrude into the client's frame of reference, not to take the client away from their own flow of experience, not to bring into the relationship the counsellor's intention to change the client, not to lead into a vocabulary that is not the client's own, not to question, probe or advise. The influence of Carl Rogers is pervasive.

> If we can provide understanding of the way the client seems to himself at this moment, he can do the rest. The therapist must lay aside his pre-occupation with diagnosis and his diagnostic shrewdness, must discard his tendency to make professional evaluations, must cease his endeavours to formulate an accurate prognoses, must give up the temptation subtly to guide the individual, and must concentrate on one purpose only; that of providing deep understanding and acceptance of his attitudes consciously held at this moment by the client as he explores step by step into the dangerous areas which he has been denying to consciousness. (p. 42)

Contrary to many people's perceptions, person-centred counselling is no soft option. It is really quite exacting both on counsellors and clients alike. There is so much to commend it, although it has to be said that, if followed in its true spirit, a number of critical issues arise when practised in a multi-agency and multi-disciplinary context. Rogers' advice and the primary preoccupation with the therapeutic relationship can lead to a very different way of working from other professionals. Its non-directive stance is at odds with more goal-orientated cognitive and behavioural approaches. Psychoanalytically trained practitioners also may look enquiringly at the place of transference and counter transference in the very congruence and authenticity of the person-centred relationship.

It is Richard Bryant-Jefferies enthusiastic commitment to the person-centred approach that drives this book so purposefully-forward. In line with his previous work, he takes hold of his thinking in this book to address a particular clinical problem – that of the plight of young binge drinkers. This is a matter of increasing public concern and all manner of solutions are being proposed. Richard Bryant-Jefferies however sees very clearly that, behind the often wild and random behaviour of such young people, there resides in many cases tales of deep discontent, fear, misery and anger.

To illustrate this, he gives us two imaginary stories – one of an 18-year-old man, the other of a 15-year-old girl. Both make compelling reading, consisting as they do of so much of the anguish and suffering that is inherent in their facing the torment of their past and current experiences. In all of this, the reader is taken well beyond the surface image of the yob and slob. And through the many moments in which the two are slowly enabled to encounter at their own pace aspects of themselves that may have lain latent and denied, they slowly find themselves with less need to binge as compulsively as they had done before.

The outcomes are positive, not perfect, not complete, but the young people less desperate, less destructive of themselves and others. If nothing else, better than ending up desolate, suicidal, abused and wretched – so clearly imagined by the author in his alternate scenarios which might well have happened had they not been received so fully in the containing presence of the counsellor.

Peter Wilson
Consultant in Child and Adolescent Mental Health
Services and Psychotherapy
Clinical Advisor to The Place To Be
Former Director of Young Minds
December 2005

Preface

The success of the preceding volumes in the *Living Therapy* series, and the continued appreciative comments received from readers and by independent reviewers,
is encouragement enough to once again extend this style into exploring the application of the person-centred approach to counselling and psychotherapy to
another challenging area of human experience – working with young binge
drinkers. Again and again people remark on how readable these books are, how
much they bring the therapeutic process alive. In particular, students of counselling and psychotherapy have remarked on how accessible the text is. Trainers
and others who are experienced in the field have indicated to me the timeliness
of a series that focuses the application of the person-centred approach to working
therapeutically with clients having particular issues. This is both heartening and
encouraging. I want the style to draw people into the narrative and for readers to
feel engaged with the characters and the therapeutic process. I want this series to
be what I would term 'an experiential read'.

As with the other volumes of the *Living Therapy* series, *Counselling Young Binge
Drinkers: person-centred dialogues* is composed of fictitious dialogues between fictitious clients Gary (aged 18 years) and Carrie (aged 15 years) and their counsellors, and between the counsellors and their supervisors. Within the dialogues are
woven the reflective thoughts and feelings of the clients, the counsellors and the
supervisors, along with boxed comments on the process and references to person-
centred theory. I do not seek to provide all the answers, or a technical manual
expounding on the right way to work with young people who are binge drinking
in a problematic manner. Rather, I want to convey something of the process of
working with representative material that can arise, so that the reader may be
stimulated into processing their own reactions, reflecting on the relevance
and effectiveness of the therapeutic responses, and thereby gaining insight into
themselves and their practice. Often it will simply lead to more questions, which
I hope will prove stimulating to the readers and encourage them to think through
their own theoretical, philosophical and ethical positions and their boundary
of competence.

Counselling Young Binge Drinkers: person-centred dialogues is intended as much
for experienced counsellors as it is for trainees. It provides real insight into what
can occur during counselling sessions. I hope it will not only raise awareness of,
and inform, person-centred practice within this context, but also contribute to

other theoretical approaches within the world of counselling, psychotherapy and the various branches of psychology. Reflections on the therapeutic process and points for discussion are included to stimulate further thought and debate. Included in this volume is material to inform the training process of counsellors and others who seek to work with young people on these issues.

I would like to draw attention to the application of the person-centred approach within education and briefly acknowledge that Carl Rogers addressed this in his books and in various papers and lectures (Rogers, 1957b, 1967b, 1969, 1977, 1980). The attitudinal values of the person-centred approach, while having therapeutic application, actually extend beyond this into all situations in which people are required to work together, where the forming of human relationships is a crucial part of a particular endeavour. I hope that this title finds its way into schools and into the hands of youth leaders, and that something of the scenarios described here could be used in educational process and awareness raising in relation to young people and alcohol use.

I hope that this book will demonstrate the value, relevance and effectiveness of this approach, providing as it does a very human response to what can be very human problems. I hope that in this volume I am able to address a range of themes that leave you, the reader, with much to reflect on and to take into your professional counselling work, whatever the setting.

Richard Bryant-Jefferies
December 2005

About the author

Richard Bryant-Jefferies qualified as a person-centred counsellor/therapist in 1994 and remains passionate about the application and effectiveness of this approach. Between early 1995 and mid-2003 Richard worked at a community drug and alcohol service in Surrey as an alcohol counsellor. Since 2003 he has worked for the Central and North West London Mental Health NHS Trust, managing the substance misuse service within the Royal Borough of Kensington and Chelsea in London. He has experience of offering both counselling and supervision in NHS, general practitioner (GP) and private settings, and has provided training through 'alcohol awareness and response' workshops. He also offers workshops based on the use of written dialogues as a contribution to continuing professional development and within training programmes. His website is: www.bryant-jefferies.freeserve.co.uk.

Richard had his first book on a counselling theme published in 2001, *Counselling the Person Beyond the Alcohol Problem* (Jessica Kingsley Publishers), providing theoretical yet practical insights into the application of the person-centred approach within the context of the 'cycle of change' model that has been widely adopted to describe the process of change in the field of addiction. Since then he was been writing for the *Living Therapy* series, producing an ongoing series of person-centred dialogues: *Problem Drinking, Time Limited Therapy in Primary Care, Counselling a Survivor of Child Sexual Abuse, Counselling a Recovering Drug User, Counselling Young People, Counselling for Progressive Disability, Relationship Counselling – Sons and their Mothers, Responding to a Serious Mental Health Problem, Person-Centred Counselling Supervision – personal and the professional, Counselling Victims of Warfare, Workplace Counselling in the NHS, Counselling for Problem Gambling, Counselling for Eating Disorders in Men, Counselling for Eating Disorders in Women* and *Counselling for Obesity.* The aim of the series is to bring the reader a direct experience of the counselling process, an exposure to the thoughts and feelings of both client and counsellor as they encounter each other on the therapeutic journey, and an insight into the value and importance of supervision.

Richard is also having published by Pen Press Ltd early in 2006 what he has entitled *A Little Book of Therapy*, offering a series of statements that clients might make during periods of stress, self-doubt or uncertainty, and affirmations to help reframe their perspective and offer opportunity for the reader to engage with the inner resources for change that they have within them.

Richard is also writing his first novel, *Dying to Live*, a story of traumatic loss, alcohol use and therapy, and has also adapted one of his books as a stage or radio play, and plans to do the same with other books in the series if the first is successful. However, he is currently seeking an opportunity for it to be recorded or staged.

Richard is keen to bring the experience of the therapeutic process, from the standpoint and application of the person-centred approach, to a wider audience. He is convinced that the principles and attitudinal values of this approach, and the emphasis it places on the therapeutic relationship, are key to helping people create greater authenticity in both themselves and their lives, leading to a fuller and more satisfying human experience. By writing fictional accounts to try and bring the therapeutic process alive, to help readers engage with the characters within the narrative – client, counsellor and supervisor – he hopes to take the reader on a journey into the counselling room. Whether we think of it as pulling back the curtains or opening a door, it is about enabling people to access what can and does occur within the therapeutic process.

Acknowledgements

Writing *Counselling Young Binge Drinkers* has required me to draw on a range of experiences, and to keep in mind the many clients whose own stories have, in different ways, contributed to what I have presented. I have seen so many adults with alcohol problems over the years whose childhoods were similar but different versions of the backgrounds of Gary and Carrie. And I have worked with people in their late teens and early twenties who have an attitude towards alcohol use that is quite devoid of any sense of its danger and the risks associated with heavy or binge drinking, until problems arise, and sometimes not even then. So, I wish to acknowledge and thank the many people that I have worked with who have shaped my thinking and feelings in writing this book.

I wish to express thanks to Robin Everall and Peter Wilson for their forewords – Robin with her emphasis on the often unrecognised or unacknowledged degrees of emotional distress present within young people and the range of self-harming behaviours that can be expressive of this, and Peter with his appreciation of the style of the book as a way of presenting therapeutic process, and his comments concerning the challenge and essential features of person-centred working.

I wish to again express my appreciation to my partner, Movena Lucas, whose past work as a substance misuse specialist within a Child and Adolescent Mental Health Service, and current role working with young people with mental health problems, provided me with further insight and kept me strongly in touch with my own thoughts and feelings towards the material being presented.

I also wish to thank Radcliffe Publishing for their continued support for the Living Therapy series which now totals 16 titles. Their belief in the ideas being presented through this series has made it all possible.

Finally, and this may sound strange, but I wish to acknowledge Gary and Carrie, the two fictional characters in this book, and thank them for taking me on a journey into myself.

'... most children, if given a reasonably normal environment, which meets their own emotional, intellectual, and social needs, have within themselves sufficient drive towards health to respond and make a comfortable adjustment to life.'

(Carl Rogers, 1939, p. 274)

Introduction

Counselling Young Binge-Drinkers: person-centred dialogues has been written with the aim of demonstrating the counsellor's application of the person-centred approach (PCA) in working with this client group which is becoming an increasing feature of our society. This theoretical approach to counselling has, at its heart, the power of the relational experience. It is this experience that I believe to be at the very heart of effective therapy, contributing to the possibility of releasing the client to realise greater potential for authentic living. The approach is widely used by counsellors working in the UK today: in a membership survey in 2001 by the British Association for Counselling and Psychotherapy, 35.6% of those responding claimed to work to the person-centred approach, while 25.4% identified themselves as psychodynamic practitioners. However, whatever the approach, it seems to me that the relationship is the key factor in contributing to a successful outcome – though this must remain a very subjective concept, for who, other than the client, can really define what experience is to be taken as a measure of a successful outcome?

Young people and alcohol

Binge drinking is an increasing phenomenon among young people. The statistics are clear. More and more young people are drinking more and more alcohol, and from an earlier age. Alcohol is an addictive and mood-altering substance. The more you drink, the greater the risk of harm. What constitutes a binge? It is defined as a daily alcohol intake that is more than twice the recommended daily safe drinking limits. Therefore a binge for men would be above eight units of alcohol, while for women it is above six units in a day.

Of course, these amounts can be easily surpassed during a heavy drinking episode. Eight units is equivalent to four pints of normal-strength beer. Many lagers are above normal strength. One measure of spirits is now a little over a unit, though some spirits are stronger still. Cocktails containing more than one type of alcoholic drink will mean that the binge-drinking level can also be reached quickly. For young people, the immediate risk from a heavy drinking episode is likely to be the effect of intoxication, although serious damage to health can and does occur. Risks to younger people are more likely to be related to physical trauma following accidents or acts of violence. Inhibitions are reduced and young people may engage in unprotected sex while under the influence of alcohol, leading to the heightened risk of unwanted pregnancy and sexually transmitted diseases. There will also be a heightened risk of alcohol poisoning; young people have smaller bodies and therefore the alcohol is likely to be more concentrated and therefore more damaging. They may also have less tolerance to alcohol, further increasing the risk of poisoning, particularly where there is no appreciation or understanding of the potency of alcohol and the effect it can have on the body and cognitive functioning. However, with young people reaching their very early 20s with 10-year histories of using alcohol, the risks of serious harm to health and of dependence are very real.

In 2004 the British Government published its *Alcohol Harm Reduction Strategy for England* (UK Government, 2004). Throughout there are references to alcohol use and young people, with particular emphasis on binge drinking and binge drinkers. In the *Interim Analytical Report* (UK Government, 2003) published the previous year, which drew together a comprehensive set of statistics concerning the impact of alcohol misuse, we read that: 'Drinkers under the age of 16 are today drinking twice as much as they did ten years ago', with alcohol being consumed by '20% of 13 year old boys and 21% of 13 year old girls; and by 49% of 15 year old boys and 45% of 15 year old girls' over the previous week. British teenagers are also among the heaviest teenage drinkers in Europe, being more likely to drink and get drunk and report alcohol-related problems than teenagers in most of the other European countries. One particular statistic stands out, that 'in the UK, more than a third of 15 years old report having been drunk at age 13 or earlier. This is true of no more than one in ten French and Italian children' (Strategy Unit, 2003, pp. 17–18).

The older teenagers and younger adults are those most likely to binge drink. Within the 16–24-year-old age group, only a quarter of women and around one in six men report never drinking more than six units (women) or eight units (men) per day. While drinking patterns change with age for many people, some will continue to binge. 'In the UK, binge drinking accounts for 40% of all drinking occasions by men and 22% by women' (Strategy Unit, 2003, pp. 20–21).

The introduction of 'alcopops' and 'ready to drink' drinks (RTDs) in 1996 was a significant development, and whilst the Strategy Unit does not offer evidence that this increased the number of young people who drink, it does highlight that this 'may have contributed to the increase in the amount drunk: between 1992 and 2001, the average amount of alcohol consumed by young people increased by 63% with approximately half of this growth first measured in the years in which RTDs were introduced' (Strategy Unit, 2004, p. 65).

Young people drink for so many reasons: peer pressure, dealing with stress from school (exams, bullying) or from home, experimentation, rebellion, coping with discomfort, to mediate the effects of drug use. In many ways the reasons are similar to those for adult alcohol use, but set in a younger, social context. For some young people the need to binge will be driven by deep psychological and emotional processes as the individual discovers that the effects make life more bearable. Often the bingeing is a symptom, an effect of something else, for instance the impact of difficult relational experiences. While directly supporting and encouraging a young person to change their drinking habit may have the desired effect of reduction, it seems more likely that the causal factors will also need to be addressed to make the likelihood of sustainable change being achieved more realistic. There is a strong case for working not just with the young person themselves. They dwell within a social world of friends, family, school or college, or work. Extending interventions to include others directly related to the young person, or who are impacting in some way on their urge, need or desire to drink, can be helpful.

Further useful statistics and information regarding young people's drinking can be found on the Alcohol Concern website (see Useful contacts, p. 189).

Access to alcohol

In the UK there is currently legislation being implemented to extend licensing hours. This has received a mixed response with evidence of growing concern among both healthcare and criminal justice professionals as to the likely impact of this change. The original idea was that extended pub opening times would reduce the phenomenon of binge drinking in the context of consuming alcohol rapidly ahead of the early closing time, and that it would reduce pressure on both criminal justice and healthcare services, with people all leaving licensed premises at a similar time.

While some commentators at the time that it was originally being suggested were expressing reservations, it is now being increasingly thought that extended licensing hours will simply encourage extended drinking and therefore further fuel the binge-drinking phenomenon.

A report from the Council of Her Majesty's Circuit Judges, which represents 600 judges, states: 'Those who routinely see the consequences of drink-fuelled violence in offences of rape, grievous bodily harm and worse on a daily basis are in no doubt that an escalation of offences of this nature will inevitably be caused by the relaxation of liquor licensing which the government has now authorised'. The Association of Chief Police Officers has reported that 'the assertion 11 pm closing leads to binge drinking is simply not supported by the evidence' (BBC News, 2005).

As far as young people are concerned, any extension to licensing hours will, in effect, extend availability to them as it does to adults. Yes, actions such as introducing identity cards to reduce the risk of serving/selling alcohol to under-age young people can help, but there is a need for the law to be strongly enforced in this area of the supply of alcohol to young people. There is also a need for more information and education, for more evidence-based treatment services, for a stronger criminal justice response to problematic drinking, greater involvement of the drinks industry in creating drinking environments that are less likely to encourage problematic drinking, and advertising that is less likely to encourage under-age drinking and binge drinking among young people (Strategy Unit, 2004).

Greater availability of alcohol, and the message that this gives is of the acceptability of 24-hour drinking, and that a society in which alcohol plays a core feature in socialising as the norm is not a problem. And, of course, it isn't a problem for many. But it is a problem for a growing number of people, particularly young people – a trend that needs to be reversed if we are to ensure that we do not become a society in which social experiencing becomes alcohol centred rather than centred in the actual social experience itself. In reality, as health and criminal justice professionals know, the more alcohol that is made available and consumed, the greater the likelihood of increasing problems which extend into the family, the workplace, health (individual and public), and society in general.

Youth matters

In the UK Government's green paper *Youth Matters*, there is recognition that young people's drinking is an area that requires addressing.

> 'Some teenagers have health problems, including chronic clinical conditions such as asthma or diabetes. In the key areas of sexual health, obesity, alcohol, volatile substance abuse and mental health, the health of adolescents is either worsening or static. This is in contrast to marked improvements in the health of younger children and older people over the last thirty years. Some young people get into bad habits such as binge drinking or drugs' (UK Government, 2005, p. 13).

Noting that as well as harming their physical health, this can lead to violence and accidents, the paper draws attention to the fact that young people are in fact the heaviest drinkers, and are more likely than all other age groups to binge drink (Health Development Agency, 2004).

Social inclusion and involvement, the encouragement of young people in active participation as citizens, greater provision and access to sports activities, and the provision of opportunity are amongst the ways forward highlighted in the Green Paper, with a number of examples cited of successful initiatives from around the UK, for instance in Oldham, where:

> 'the Youth Offending Service, Connexions and the Drugs and Alcohol Action Team are co-located in a Connexions branded one stop shop. They are managed under the umbrella of Positive Steps Oldham, a charitable trust. The trust also delivers the positive activities scheme during school holidays. Oldham was cited in the Audit Commission's report on youth justice (2004) as an exemplar of inter-agency, co-located working' (UK Government, 2005, p. 61).

It is likely that such centres will become more widely established, offering a positive young person-centred service. Such 'one stop shop' initiatives may be extended, to include other treatment and social care services on a sessional basis, reducing the stigmatising effect of having to attend more traditional services within separate locations.

The green paper offers an opportunity for consultation on a number of proposals designed to develop young people into responsible citizens within the community. The aim is to encourage a more integrated response in developing and commissioning services for young people, with far greater involvement from young people within these processes. Without doubt, a more integrated response is required, and involvement from young people is absolutely necessary. Young people do need opportunities to develop social lives that are less centred around binge drinking, offering the possibility of making choices that are less harmful to themselves and others. Time will tell, however, whether such initiatives will be enough to offset the increased availability of alcohol through the Government's reform of the licensing laws.

One note of caution is that there is a strong emphasis on the use of consumerism (whether entertainment or goods) to deflect young people from problematic behaviour. And while sports activities, schemes to offer training and pathways into work, opportunities for volunteering and encouraging citizenship are emphasised, perhaps there might also need to be scope to encourage young people to take greater interest in nature, the environment, in experiences that are less frenetic, that enable a sense of slowing down in order to have time to experience feelings rather than be driven from experience to experience, from behaviour to behaviour.

Referral pathways and access to counselling

One of the key aspects of the provision of services for young people with alcohol problems is that there need to be very clear referral pathways for young people to access services. For this to be effective, there has to be 'joined-up thinking' across service provision, offering an informed and seamless system of care and treatment pathways. Problematic alcohol use needs to be identified at the earliest opportunity, and having been identified can then be responded to directly or the young people referred to, or encouraged to attend, a specialist service

From the teacher at school, to parents, there is a need for an understanding of how best to respond, and to whom a young person should be referred for more specialist advice, support or, indeed, treatment. Many drug action teams (DATs) are now drug and alcohol action teams (DAATs), and are seeking to ensure that services that do not directly carry a specialism in alcohol, but that do specialise in working with young people, are more fully aware of alcohol issues and have the skills to offer screening and to identify problems, and have the necessary systems in place for referral on. Many DATs and DAATs are now actively formulating and implementing common screening and assessment form procedures across services working with young people, services that are not specialists in alcohol (or drug) use but that will be able to offer initial interventions and initiate referral on where required.

In some areas in the UK there are specialist alcohol services for young people, in other areas the services may be simply part of adult services, or handled through child and adolescent mental health services (CAMHS). But these are more likely to be for young people with particularly serious problems. The Connexions network also caters for young people with alcohol problems, and there are many non-statutory services providing interventions and support, although this varies around the country.

There has been a general recognition that, for young people, alcohol treatment generally needs to be in a wider social context and not simply an alcohol-centred intervention. Response can be as much concerned with helping the young person to cope with their lives, with familial, school or relational problems in order to reduce their need to rely on alcohol and its effects, or to review their social lives and the choices they have been making, and the associated risks. As with young people with drug problems, the emphasis in response to young binge drinkers often needs to be upon reintegrating the child into educational processes, training, work and, most significantly of course, back into a functional family system.

In addition to the above, young binge drinkers may require support for other difficulties, whether directly or indirectly associated. There could be other drug use, with the alcohol being used to manage the highs from, for instance, stimulant use. Perhaps more dangerously, it might be being used in combination with cannabis or heroin, adding to the suppressant effect and exacerbating the risk of overdose. There may be mental health problems present, the alcohol either causing problems, or being used by the young person to manage their own symptoms. There may be familial and social difficulties as well, requiring a specific set of interventions to help reduce the young person's perceived need to turn to alcohol.

Not all young people will want 'counselling' in a traditional sense. It can seem strange to some young people who may prefer a more informal chat with someone that they respect, or who they feel understands. Hence the importance, alluded to earlier, of ensuring that other professionals or people working in the voluntary sector with young people have the necessary knowledge to engage with them on the topic of binge drinking.

Counselling young people

Counselling young people is becoming more widespread in our society. Since the 1960s, counselling has become more of a feature in schools, and youth counselling services have become established in both the voluntary and statutory sectors of health and social care. With this have come the many challenges associated with forming a therapeutic relationship with young people, and the seemingly difficult legal landscape associated with the young person's right to confidentiality and their competence to consent to treatment. The legal position has been usefully discussed by Jenkins (2002) who argues the need for counsellors and psychotherapists working with children and young people to be familiar with the background to the establishing of the Gillick principle and the ensuing case law, including the *Fraser Guidelines*. It is not the intention in this volume to explore this; the reader is, however, encouraged to undertake their own research on this important topic.

Let us turn to the therapeutic relationship with young people. What are the factors that contribute to a successful therapeutic experience? An interesting piece of research into adolescent perspectives on the therapeutic alliance has suggested that the factors of 'therapeutic environment . . . the climate or "ambience" within which the therapist and client functioned which set the tone for what was to follow'; 'the uniqueness of the therapeutic relationship . . . comprised of an egalitarian foundation, a sense of trust and respect, and a view that the therapist was a special friend'; and certain 'therapist characteristics . . . a sense that the therapist was authentic, open and sincerely cared . . . manifested through a genuine emotional response that was described as sensitive, sympathetic and kind' are of primary importance (Everall and Paulson, 2002, pp. 81–3). These attitudinal qualities bear a close resemblance to those posited by Rogers as fundamental conditions for constructive personality change. Indeed, the authors of this study comment that 'the development of a therapeutic alliance with adolescents appears to be consistent with the research on the therapeutic triad of empathy, genuineness and respect (Rogers, 1957a). Warmth and empathy were clearly identified by our participants who used identical words that Rogers used to identify the core conditions' (Everall and Paulson, 2002, pp. 84–5).

However, the study also highlighted negative experiences, and the adolescents referred to the relationship with the therapist 'being similar to other interactions with adults in terms of a power differential and was identified as having an authoritarian foundation'. The negative impact of the therapist taking the role of 'expert', of not listening to what the young person was saying about their experiences, and feeling that they were not being treated respectfully, were emphasised. In particular, the authors of the study report 'lack of respect [that] resulted in withdrawal from engagement' (Everall and Paulson, 2002, p. 85).

The fact that the young people saw the counselling relationship as 'special' and the therapist as 'a special friend' offers valuable insight into the inner world of the young clients. They indicated how important this was, and what a contrast to their usual experience of being in relationship with adults. This contrast was reported as being difficult at first, the client perhaps being wary, not sure what was going on, finding their expectations challenged and taking time to settle into a feeling of trust towards the therapist.

It seems highly likely that for effective counselling of young people there needs to be an adaptation in style, a readiness and willingness by the counsellor to be open, to really want to be psychologically alongside the young person, to enable that young person to feel at ease and to share whatever is present for them. I have certainly come across counsellors who participate in other activities with the client, chatting with them as they do so, encouraging the client to share in a more conversational form of therapeutic encounter.

This is not a licence for 'anything goes'. The therapist remains disciplined, but open to the means of communication that most effectively help them build a therapeutic alliance with the client. For the person-centred counsellor, the intention will be to be open to direction from the client, to be prepared to learn what most helps that young person gain what they need from the therapeutic experience.

Gaylin highlights the particular importance of therapist congruence when working with young people. He suggests that:

> 'Before they entrust adults with their deeply personal thoughts and feelings they need to believe the adults are worthy of that trust. Children are masters of nonverbal communication – more so than adults – and thus can sense deception and guile. Simply put, young people of all ages demand congruence in their therapists if therapy is to be effective' (Gaylin, 2001, p. 124).

I would suggest that as adults get real with young people – genuinely and authentically, with clear self-awareness and openness to their own experiencing – then there is a much higher likelihood that young people will feel encouraged to become more real themselves, more openly present and able to engage more fully, and with clarity of awareness, with the range of experiencing that is open to them as human beings.

More recently, a scoping review of counselling children and young people has been produced (Harris and Pattison, 2004) which was commissioned by the British Association for Counselling and Psychotherapy (BACP) in order to add to the research base in counselling children and young people. The review looks at a variety of presenting issues in counselling children and young people, including behavioural and conduct disorders; emotional problems including anxiety, depression and post-traumatic stress; medical illness; school-related issues; self-harming practices and sexual abuse.

The person-centred approach

The person-centred approach (PCA) was formulated by Carl Rogers, and references are made to his ideas within the text of this book. However, it will be helpful for readers who are unfamiliar with this way of working to have an appreciation of its theoretical base.

Rogers proposed that certain conditions, when present within a therapeutic relationship, would enable the client to develop towards what he termed 'fuller functionality'. Over a number of years he refined these ideas, which he defined as 'the necessary and sufficient conditions for constructive personality change'. These he described as:

1 two persons are in psychological contact
2 the first, whom we shall term the client, is in a state of incongruence, being vulnerable or anxious

3　the second person, whom we shall term the therapist, is congruent or integrated in the relationship
4　the therapist experiences unconditional positive regard for the client
5　the therapist experiences an empathic understanding of the client's internal frame of reference and endeavours to communicate this experience to the client
6　the communication to the client of the therapist's empathic understanding and unconditional positive regard is to a minimal degree achieved (Rogers, 1957a, p. 96).

Contact

The first necessary and sufficient condition given for constructive personality change is that of 'two person being in psychological contact'. However, although he later published this as simply 'contact' (Rogers, 1959), it is suggested (Wyatt and Saunders, 2002, p. 6) that this was actually written in 1953–54. Wyatt and Saunders quote Rogers as defining contact in the following terms: 'Two persons are in psychological contact, or have the minimum essential relationship when each makes a perceived or subceived difference in the experiential field of the other' (Rogers, 1959, p. 207). A recent exploration of the nature of psychological contact from a person-centred perspective is given by Warner (2002).

There is much to reflect on when considering a definition of 'contact' or 'psychological contact'. We might think of this in terms of whether the therapist's presence is, to some minimal degree, impacting on the awareness of the client; that, if you like, the field of awareness of the client is affected by the therapist. And, of course, the opposite holds, that the client's presence is also impacting on the field of awareness of the counsellor. It is the first condition given, and arguably the foundation for therapy. It does not necessarily mean, however, that client and therapist are sitting together in the same room, hence telephone and Internet counselling also involve contact. Whatever the situation, contact or psychological contact is indicated by each having awareness of the other.

In terms of therapeutic significance, are there degrees of contact? Is it true that contact is a matter of being either present or not, or is there a kind of continuum of contact, with greater or lesser degrees or depths of contact? It seems to me that it is both, that rather like the way that light may be regarded as either a particle or a wave, contact may be seen as a specific state of being, or as a process, depending upon what the perceiver is seeking to measure or observe. If I am trying to observe or measure whether there is contact, then my answer will be in terms of 'yes' or 'no'. If I am seeking to determine the degree to which contact exists, then the answer will be along a continuum. In other words, from the moment of minimal contact there is contact, but that contact can then extend, as more aspects of the client become present within the therapeutic relationship which, itself, may at times reach moments of increasing depth.

Empathy

Rogers defined empathy as meaning 'entering the private perceptual world of the other ... being sensitive, moment by moment, to the changing felt meanings which flow in this other person ... It means sensing meanings of which he or she is scarcely aware, but not trying to uncover totally unconscious feelings' (Rogers, 1980, p. 142). It is a very delicate process, and it provides a foundation block to effective person-centred therapy. The counsellor's role is primarily to establish empathic rapport and communicate empathic understanding to the client. This latter point is vital. Empathic understanding only has therapeutic value where it is communicated to the client.

I would like to add another comment regarding empathy. There is so much more to empathy than simply letting the client know what you understand from what they have communicated. It is also, and perhaps more significantly, the actual *process* of listening to a client, of attending – facial expression, body language, and presence – that is being offered and communicated and received *at the time that the client is speaking, at the time that the client is experiencing what is present for them*. It is, for the client, the knowing that, in the moment of an experience, the counsellor is present and striving to be an understanding companion.

Unconditional positive regard

Within the therapeutic relationship the counsellor seeks to maintain an attitude of unconditional positive regard towards the client and all that they disclose. This is not 'agreeing with', it is simply warm acceptance of the fact that the client is being how they need or choose to be. Rogers wrote, 'when the therapist is experiencing a positive, acceptant attitude towards whatever the client *is* at that moment, therapeutic movement or change is more likely to occur' (Rogers, 1980, p. 116). Mearns and Thorne suggest that:

> 'Unconditional positive regard is the label given to the fundamental attitude of the person-centred counsellor towards her client. The counsellor who holds this attitude deeply values the humanity of her client and is not deflected in that valuing by any particular client behaviours. The attitude manifests itself in the counsellor's consistent acceptance of and enduring warmth towards her client' (Mearns and Thorne, 1988, p. 59).

Both Bozarth (1998) and Wilkins assert that 'unconditional positive regard is the curative factor in person-centred therapy' (Bozarth and Wilkins, 2001, p.vii). It is perhaps worth speculatively drawing these two statements together. We might then suggest that the unconditional positive regard experienced and conveyed by the counsellor, and received by the client as an expression of the counsellor's valuing of their client's humanity, has a curative role in the therapeutic process. We might then add that this may be the case more specifically for those individuals who have been affected by a lack of unconditional warmth and prizing in their lives.

Congruence

Congruence is a state of being that Rogers has also described in terms of 'real-ness', 'transparency', 'genuineness', 'authenticity'. Indeed, Rogers wrote that '... genuineness, realness or congruence ... this means that the therapist is openly being the feelings and attitudes that are flowing within at the moment ... the term transparent catches the flavour of this condition' (Rogers, 1980, p. 116). Putting this into the therapeutic setting, we can say that 'congruence is the state of being of the counsellor when her outward responses to her client con-sistently match the inner feelings and sensations which she has in relation to her client' (Mearns and Thorne, 1999, p. 84). Interestingly, Rogers makes the follow-ing comment in his interview with Richard Evans. that with regard to the three conditions, 'first, and most important, is therapist congruence or genuineness ... one description of what it means to be congruent in a given moment is to be aware of what's going on in your experiencing at that moment, to be acceptant towards that experience, to be able to voice it if it's appropriate, and to express it in some behavioural way' (Evans, 1975).

I would suggest that any congruent expression by the counsellor of their feel-ings or reactions has to emerge through the process of being in therapeutic rela-tionship with the client. Indeed, the condition indicates that the therapist is congruent or integrated into the relationship. This indicates the significance of the relationship. Being congruent is a disciplined way of being and not an open door to endless self-disclosure. Congruent expression is perhaps most appropriate and therapeutically valuable where it is informed by the existence of an empathic understanding of the client's inner world, and is offered in a climate of a genuine warm acceptance towards the client. Having said that, it is reasonable to suggest that, taking Rogers' comment quoted above that regarding congruence as 'most important', we might suggest that unless the therapist is congruent in themselves and in the relationship, then their empathy and unconditional positive regard would be at risk of not being authentic or genuine.

Another view, however, would be that it is in some way false to distinguish or rather seek to separate out the three 'core conditions', that they exist together as a whole, mutually dependent on each other's presence in order to ensure that therapeutic relationship is established.

Perception

There is also the sixth condition, of which Rogers wrote:

> 'The final condition ... is that the client perceives, to a minimal degree, the acceptance and empathy which the therapist experiences for him. Unless some communication of these attitudes has been achieved, then such attitudes do not exist in the relationship as far as the client is concerned, and the thera-peutic process could not, by our hypothesis, be initiated' (Rogers, 1957a).

It is interesting that he uses the words 'minimal degree', suggesting that the client does not need to fully perceive the fullness of the empathy and unconditional positive regard present within, and communicated by, the counsellor. A glimpse warmly accepted, accurately heard and empathically understood is enough to have positive, therapeutic effect although logically one might think that the more that is perceived, the greater the therapeutic impact. But if it is a matter of intensity and accuracy, then for a client the experience of a vitally important fragment of their inner world being empathically understood and warmly accepted may be more significant to them, and more therapeutically significant, than a great deal being heard less accurately and with a weaker sense of therapist understanding and acceptance. The communication of the counsellor's empathy, congruence and unconditional positive regard, received by the client, creates the conditions for a process of constructive personality change.

The vital importance of contact and of the client perceiving the presence of the counsellor's unconditional positive regard and empathic understanding towards him cannot be overstated. Conditions one and six of the necessary and sufficient conditions for constructive personality change as formulated by Rogers have become a focus for theoretical discussion and debate, and rightly so. While they may not represent 'core conditions' insofar as the attitudinal qualities of empathy, congruence and unconditional positive regard are concerned, they provide the relational framework through which these attitudinal qualities can have therapeutic value and effect. Indeed, without the presence of contact and perception as described by Rogers (1957a, 1959), there would be no relational framework for the therapeutic process to occur. This leaves us with the position that perhaps conditions one (contact) and six (perception) are in reality the 'primary core conditions' as they define the presence of a relationship. Then, unconditional positive regard and empathic understanding might be seen to define the quality of the relationship, while client incongruence and counsellor congruence define the state of being brought into the relationship. Taken together, there emerges the existence of what we might then term a 'person-centred therapeutic relationship'.

Relationship is key

The PCA regards the relationship that counsellors have with their clients, and the attitude that they hold within that relationship, to be key factors. Cooper (2004) has reviewed findings from a range of studies from researchers and theorists to argue that 'there is growing support for a relationship-orientated approach to therapeutic practice' (Cooper, p. 452). Among the evidence that he cites is a vast review of research on the therapeutic relationship commissioned in 1999 by the American Psychological Association Division of Psychotherapy Task Force, which, citing Norcross (2002b), was the largest ever review of research on the therapeutic relationship with its distillation of evidence coming to over 400 pages. To quote from what Cooper has to say in his paper: 'Its main conclusion was that "The therapy relationship ... makes

substantial and consistent contributions to psychotherapy outcome independent of the specific type of treatment"' (Steering Committee, 2002, p. 441).
(The 'therapy relationship' is defined here as 'the feelings and attitudes that
therapist and client have towards one another, and the manner in which these
are expressed' (Norcross, 2002a, p. 7).)

Further conclusions Cooper (2004) cites from this study include, 'Practice and
treatment guidelines should explicitly address therapist behaviours and qualities
that promote a facilitative therapy relationship' and 'Efforts to promulgate practice guidelines or evidence-based lists of effective psychotherapy without including the therapy relationship are seriously incomplete and potentially misleading
on both clinical and empirical grounds' (Steering Committee, 2002, p. 441). Also
the recommendation is made that practitioners should 'make the creation and
cultivation of a therapy relationship ... a primary aim in the treatment of
patients' (Steering Committee, 2002, p. 442).

In my experience, many adult psychological difficulties develop out of life
experiences that involve problematic, conditional or abusive relational experiences. This can be centred in childhood or later in life, and in this volume we
focus on the development of binge drinking in young people. What is significant
is that the individual is left, through relationships that have a negative conditioning effect, with a distorted perception of themselves and their potential as a
person. Patterns are established in early life, bringing their own particular problems, but they can be exacerbated by conditional and psychologically damaging
experiences later in life, that in some cases will have a resonance to what has
occurred in the past, exacerbating the effects still further.

An oppressive experience can impact on a child's confidence in themselves,
leaving them anxious, uncertain and moving towards establishing patterns of
thought, feeling and behaviour associated with the developing concept of themselves typified by 'I am weak and cannot expect to be treated any differently',
'I just have to accept this attitude towards me, what can I do to change anything?'. These psychological conclusions may rest on patterns of thinking and
feeling already established; perhaps the person was bullied at school, or experienced rejection in the home. They may have had a lifetime of stress, or it may be
a relatively new experience; either way, a mode of thinking may develop typified
by 'it's normal to feel stressed, you just keep going, whatever it takes'.

The result is a conditioned sense of self, with the individual then thinking,
feeling and acting in ways that enable them to maintain their self-beliefs and
meanings within their learned or adapted concept of self. This is then lived out,
with the person seeking to satisfy what they have come to believe about themselves: needing to care either because it has been normalised, or in order to
prove to themselves and the world that they are a 'good' person. They will
need to maintain this conditioned sense of self and the sense of satisfaction that
this gives them when it is lived out, because they have developed such a strong
identity with it. Binge drinking can be one factor in maintaining a particular
sense of self, or in creating a new one in order to escape from discomfort.

The term 'conditions of worth' applies to the conditioning mentioned previously that is frequently present in childhood, and at other times in life, when a

person experiences that their worth is conditional on their doing something or behaving in a certain way. This is usually to satisfy someone else's needs, and can be contrary to the client's own sense of what would be a satisfying experience. The values of others become a feature of the individual's structure of self. The person moves away from being true to themselves, learning instead to remain 'true' to their conditioned sense of worth. This state of being in the client is challenged by the person-centred therapist by offering them unconditional positive regard and warm acceptance. Such a therapist, by genuinely offering these therapeutic attitudes, provides the client with an opportunity to be exposed to what may be a new experience or one that in the past they have dismissed, preferring to stay with that which matches and therefore reinforces their conditioned sense of worth and sense of self.

By offering someone a non-judgemental, warm and accepting, and authentic relationship (perhaps a kind of 'therapeutic love'), that person can grow into a fresh sense of self in which their potential as a person can become more fulfilled. It enables them to liberate themselves from the constraints of patterns of conditioning. Such an experience fosters an opportunity for the client to redefine themselves as they experience the presence of the therapist's congruence, empathy and unconditional positive regard. This process can take time. Often the personality change necessary to sustain a shift away from what have been termed 'conditions of worth' may require a lengthy period of therapeutic work, bearing in mind that the person may be struggling to unravel a sense of self that has been developed, sustained and reinforced for many decades of life. Of course, where it has been established more recently, then less time may be necessary.

Actualising tendency

A crucial feature or factor in this process of 'constructive personality change' is the presence of what Rogers (Rogers, 1986) termed 'the actualising tendency', a tendency towards fuller and more complete personhood with an associated greater fulfilment of their potentialities. The role of the person-centred counsellor is to provide the facilitative climate within which this tendency can work constructively. The 'therapist trusts the actualizing tendency of the client and truly believes that the client who experiences the freedom of a fostering psychological climate will resolve his or her own problems' (Bozarth, 1998, p. 4). This is fundamental to the application of the person-centred approach. Rogers (1986, p. 198) wrote:

> 'The person-centred approach is built on a basic trust in the person ... [It] depends on the actualizing tendency present in every living organism – the tendency to grow, to develop, to realize its full potential. This way of being trusts the constructive directional flow of the human being towards a more complex and complete development. It is this directional flow that we aim to release'.

Having said this, we must also acknowledge that for some people, or at certain stages, rather than producing a liberating experience, there will instead be a tendency to maintain the status quo. Perhaps the fear of change, the uncertainty or the implications of change are such that the person prefers to maintain the known, the certain. In a sense, there is a liberation from the imperative to change and grow which may bring temporary – and perhaps permanent – relief for the person. The actualising tendency may work through the part of the person that needs relief from change, enhancing its presence for the period of time that the person experiences a need to maintain this. The person-centred therapist will not try to move the person from this place or state. It is to be accepted, warmly and unconditionally. And, of course, sometimes in the moment of acceptance the person is enabled to question whether that really is how they want to be. But that is another part of the process.

Configuration within self

It is of value to draw attention, at this point, to the notion of 'configurations within self'. Configurations within self (Mearns and Thorne, 2000) are discrete sets of thoughts, feelings and behaviours that develop through the experience of life. They emerge in response to a range of experiences, including the process of introjection and the symbolisation of experiences, as well as in response to dissonant self-experience within the person's structure of self. They can also exist in what Mearns terms '"growthful" and "not for growth", configurations' (Mearns and Thorne, 2000, pp. 114–16), each offering a focus for the actualising tendency, the former seeking an expansion into new areas of experience with all that that brings, the latter seeking to energise the status quo and to block change because of its potential for disrupting the current order within the structure of self. The actualising tendency may not always manifest through growth or developmental change. It can also manifest through periods of stabilisation and stability, or a wanting to get away from something. The self is seen as a constellation of configurations, with the individual moving between them and living through them in response to experience.

Mearns suggests that these 'parts' or 'configurations' interrelate 'like a family, with an individual variety of dynamics'. As within any 'system', change in one area will impact on the functioning of the system. He therefore comments that:

> 'When the interrelationship of configurations changes, it is not that we are left with something entirely new: we have the same "parts" as before, but some which may have been subservient before are stronger, others which were judged adversely are accepted, some which were in self-negating conflict have come to respect each other, and overall the parts have achieved constructive integration with the energy release which arises from such fusion' (Mearns and Thorne, 1999, pp. 147–8).

The growing acceptance of the configurations, their own fluidity and movement within the self-structure, the increased, open and more accurate communication between the parts, is, perhaps, another way of considering the weaving together of the threads of experience to which Rogers refers (1967a, p. 158).

In terms of these ideas, we can anticipate clients containing, within themselves, particular configurations with which certain drinking patterns and related behaviours are associated. A configuration may have developed that associates the effects of binge drinking with a sense of autonomy, of being able to express oneself in a particular way. Alcohol use can enable feelings to emerge and be expressed, as much as it can cause them to be suppressed. Drinking alcohol may allow a particular configuration to assume dominance. If that configuration then assumes a certain psychological primacy, the associated drinking may also take a similar position in the person's life.

There may also be 'not for bingeing' configurations as well, of course, or a configuration may develop or emerge into primacy that is made up of the behaviours, thoughts and feelings associated with the client's establishment of a different perspective towards themselves expressed through a different drinking pattern, or a non-drinking pattern. Understanding the configurational nature of ourselves enables us to understand why we are triggered into certain thoughts, feelings and behaviours, and how they group together, serving a particular experiential purpose for the person. And where binge drinking is one of the associated behaviours of a configuration, its emergence into awareness will increase the likelihood that the behaviour will follow. As we see more and more young people developing binge-drinking patterns, and from an earlier age, and particularly at ages where developmental processes are still very much present and the young person is developing a sense of themselves in preparation for adulthood, the psychological impact may be more profound, with configurations within the self developing and including the tendency to binge drink at a fundamental level within the self-structure.

From this theoretical perspective we can argue that the person-centred counsellor's role is essentially facilitative. Creating the therapeutic climate of empathic understanding, unconditional positive regard and authenticity creates a relational experience that encourages the client to move into a more fluid state with more openness to their own experience and the discovery of a capacity towards a fuller actualising of their potential.

Relationship re-emphasised

In addressing these factors, the therapeutic relationship is central. A therapeutic approach such as a person-centred one affirms that it is not what you do so much as *how you are* with your client that is therapeutically significant, and this 'how you are' has to be received by the client. Gaylin (2001, p. 103) highlights the importance of client perception: 'If clients believe that their therapist is working on their behalf – if they perceive caring and understanding – then therapy is likely to be successful. It is the condition of attachment and the perception of connection that have the power to release the faltered actualization of the self'. He goes on to stress how 'we all need to feel connected, prized – loved', describing human beings as 'a species born into mutual interdependence' and that there 'can be no self outside the context of others. Loneliness is dehumanizing and isolation anathema to the human condition. The relationship', he suggests 'is what psychotherapy is all about'.

Love is an important word though not necessarily one often used to describe therapeutic relationship. Patterson, however, gives a valuable definition of love as it applies to the person-centred therapeutic process. He writes, 'we define love as an attitude that is expressed through empathic understanding, respect and compassion, acceptance, and therapeutic genuineness, or honesty and openness towards others' (Patterson, 2000, p. 315). We all need love, but most of all we need it during our developmental period of life. The same author affirms that 'whilst love is important throughout life for the well-being of the individual, it is particularly important, indeed absolutely necessary, for the survival of the infant and for providing the basis for the normal psychological development of the individual' (Patterson, 2000, pp. 314–15).

In a previous volume in this series I used the analogy of treating a wilting plant (Bryant-Jefferies, 2003, p. 12). We can spray it with some specific herbicide or pesticide to eradicate a perceived disease that may be present in that plant, and that may be enough. But perhaps the true cause of the disease is that the plant is located in harsh surroundings, perhaps too much sun and not enough water, poor soil, near other plants that it finds difficulty in surviving so close to. Maybe by offering the plant a healthier environment that will facilitate greater nourishment according to the needs of the plant, we can help it become the strong, healthy plant it has the potential to be. Yes, the chemical intervention may also be helpful, but if the true causes of the diseases are environmental – essentially the plant's relationship with that which surrounds it – then it won't actually achieve sustainable growth. We may not be able to transplant it, but we can provide water, nutrients and maybe shade from a fierce sun. Therapy, it seems to me, exists to provide this healthy environment within which the wilting client can begin the process of receiving the nourishment (in the form of healthy relational experience) that can enable them, in time, to become a more fully functioning person.

Diagnosis

It is interesting to consider 'binge drinking' and alcohol problems in relation to diagnosis. The person-centred view of diagnosis generally regards it as a language associated with a medical model of working, and not always necessarily helpful or indeed descriptive beyond the person's behaviour or a set of symptoms. It may not be the cause. This is certainly true regarding binge drinking. The reasons why an individual develops a binge-drinking pattern will be unique to them, will be the result of their own uniquely internalised meanings flowing from their own individual experiences, and their own psychological and behavioural needs.

Is binge drinking among young people a medical or social problem? It can cause medical and social problems, but what drives the need to binge? As we know, the causes are many; some may be more psychologically driven by traumatic or difficult experiences, for others it is simply the thing to do. What is perhaps concerning is that as binge drinking becomes increasingly the established culture, more young people are at risk of adopting it without thought; it becomes a part of the societal norm marking the adolescent transition into adulthood. This cannot be positive. If anything needs a diagnosis, it may be society more than the individual young people themselves, whose drinking choices are simply the symptom.

While a particular set of symptoms may be usefully grouped under a heading, the risk is that the diagnosis assumes that the person has a set 'illness' that will be resolved by a specific 'treatment'. Binge drinking in young people is not an illness, but a symptom of other processes, indeed perhaps of a much wider societal malaise. We might even go so far as to suggest this is true for problem drinkers of all ages except, perhaps, where chemical changes as a result of the continued alcohol use have left the person chemically dependent on alcohol. Where the problem is more of a psychological dependence, then it is the psychological factors that need addressing. The alcohol problem is secondary, and probably to the client a coping mechanism, a solution more than a problem.

I have referred elsewhere (Bryant-Jefferies, 2003) to the debate as to whether diagnosis can necessarily be trusted and empirical when it comes to mental health factors, drawing attention to Bozarth (2002) who refers to his own studies of particular diagnostic concepts which do not evidence the clustering of symptoms in a meaningful way (Bozarth 1998), and to those of others in relation to schizophrenia (Slade and Cooper, 1979; Bentall, 1990), depression (Weiner, 1989; Hallett, 1990), agoraphobia (Hallam, 1983), borderline personality disorder (Kutchins and Kirk, 1997) and panic disorder (Hallam, 1989). Perspectives on psychopathology have more recently been offered by Joseph and Worsley (2005), drawing together a number of writers and practitioners to address mental health themes from a person-centred perspective, and seeking to offer a positive psychology of mental health.

Rogers also questioned the value of psychological diagnosis. He argued that it could place the client's locus of value firmly outside themselves and definitely within the diagnosing 'expert', leaving the client at risk of developing tendencies of dependence and expectation that the 'expert' will have the responsibility of improving the client's situation (Rogers, 1951, p. 223). He also formulated the following propositional statements (pp. 221–3):

'Behaviour is caused, and the psychological cause of behaviour is a certain perception or a way of perceiving.'

'The client is the only one who has the potentiality of knowing fully the dynamics of his perceptions and his behaviour.'

'In order for behaviour to change, a change in perception must be *experienced*. Intellectual knowledge cannot substitute for this.'

'The constructive forces which bring about altered perception, reorganization of self, and relearning, reside primarily in the client, and probably cannot come from outside.'

'Therapy is basically the experiencing of the inadequacies in old ways of perceiving, the experiencing of new and more accurate and adequate perceptions, and the recognition of significant relationship between perceptions.'

'In a very meaningful and accurate sense, therapy *is* diagnosis, and this diagnosis is a process which goes on in the experience of the client, rather than in the intellect of the clinician.'

Vincent has drawn together some valuable passages from Rogers in relation to the question of diagnosis, emphasising that '*therapist* diagnosis, evaluation and prognosis clearly do not respect the inner resources of *clients*, and their potential and capacity for self-direction, as there is an obvious implication that actually the therapist, not the client, knows best' (Vincent, 2005, p.53). He then quotes a passage from Rogers from his earlier days, a statement that stands the test of time, sounding with great clarity an essential person-centred perspective on this issue:

'If we can provide understanding of the way the client seems to himself at this moment, he can do the rest. The therapist must lay aside his pre-occupation with diagnosis and his diagnostic shrewdness, must discard his tendency to make professional evaluations, must cease his endeavours to formulate an accurate prognosis, must give up the temptation subtly to guide the individual, and must concentrate on one purpose only; that of providing deep understanding and acceptance of his attitudes consciously held at this moment by the client as he explores step by step into the dangerous areas which he has been denying to consciousness' (Rogers, 1946, p. 420).

The process of change from a person-centred perspective

Rogers was interested in understanding the process of change, what it was like, how it occurred and what experiences it brought to those involved – client and therapist. At different points he explored this. Embleton Tudor *et al* (2004) point to a model consisting of 12 steps identified in 1942 (Rogers, 1942) and to his two later chapters on this topic (Rogers, 1951), and finally the seven-stage model (1967a). He wrote of 'initially looking for elements which would mark or characterize change itself'. However, he summarised what he experienced from his enquiry and research into the process of change: 'individuals move, I began to see, not from fixity or homeostasis through change to a new fixity, though such a process is indeed possible. But much the more significant continuum is from fixity to changingness, from rigid structure to flow, from stasis to process.

I formed the tentative hypothesis that perhaps the qualities of the client's expression at any one point might indicate his position on this continuum, where he stood in the process of change' (Rogers, 1967a, p. 131).

Change, then, involves a movement from fixity to greater fluidity, from a rigid set of attitudes and behaviours to a greater openness to experience, variety and diversity. Change might be seen as having a certain liberating quality, a freeing up of the human being – heart, mind, emotions – so that the person experiences themselves less as a fixed object and more of a conscious process. For the client who is seeking to resolve issues associated with problematic binge-drinking behaviours, part of this process will involve a loosening of their identity that is strongly connected to the image they have of themself linked to their drinking, or of the underlying feelings and experiences that may be driving the urge to binge to deal with emotional and psychological discomfort. Until this is 'unfixed', if you like, it would seem reasonable to conclude that sustainable change might be extremely difficult to achieve.

The list below is taken from Rogers' summary of the process, indicating the changes that people will show.

1 'This process involves a loosening of feelings.
2 This process involves a change in the manner of experiencing.
3 This process involves a shift from incongruence to congruence.
4 This process involves a change in the manner in which, and the extent to which the individual is able and willing to communicate himself in a receptive climate.
5 This process involves a loosening of the cognitive maps of experience.
6 There is a change in the individual's relationship to his problem.
7 There is a change in the individual's manner of relating' (Rogers, 1967a, pp. 156–8).

This is a very partial overview; the chapter in which he describes the process of change has much more detail and should be read in order to gain a clear grasp of the process as a whole, as well as the distinctive features of each stage as he saw it. Tudor and Worrall summarise this process in the following terms: 'a movement from fixity to fluidity, from closed to open, from tight to loose, and from afraid to accepting' (2004, p. 47).

In Rogers' description, he makes the point that there were several types of process by which personality changes and that the process he described is one that is 'set in motion when the individual experiences himself as being fully received' (Rogers, 1967a, p. 151). Does this process apply to all psychotherapies? Rogers indicated that more data were needed, adding that 'perhaps therapeutic approaches which place great stress on the cognitive and little on the emotional aspects of experience may set in motion an entirely different process of change'. In terms of whether this process of change would generally be viewed as desirable and would move the person in a valued direction, Rogers expressed the view that the valuing of a particular process of change was linked to social value judgements made by individuals and cultures. He pointed out that the process of change that he described could be avoided, simply by people 'reducing or avoiding those relationships in which the individual is fully received as he is' (Rogers, 1967a, p. 151).

Rogers also took the view that change was unlikely to be rapid, making the point that many clients enter the therapeutic process at stage two, and leave at stage four, having gained enough during that period to feel satisfied. He suggested it would be 'very rare, if ever, that a client who fully exemplified stage one would move to a point where he full exemplified stage seven', and that if this did occur 'it would involve a matter of years' (Rogers, 1967a, pp. 155–6). He wrote of how, at the outset, the threads of experience are discerned and understood separately by the client but as the process of change takes place, they move into 'the flowing peak moments of therapy in which all these threads become inseparably woven together'. He continues: 'in the new experiencing with immediacy which occurs at such moments, feeling and cognition interpenetrate, self is subjectively present in the experience, volition is simply the subjective following of a harmonious balance of organismic direction. Thus, as the process reaches this point the person becomes a unity of flow, of motion. He has changed, but what seems most significant, he has become an integrated process of changingness' (Rogers, 1967a, p. 158).

It conjures up images of flowing movement, perhaps we should say purposeful flowing movement, as being the essence of the human condition, a state that we each have the potential to become or to realise. Is it something we generate or develop out of fixity, or does it exist within us all as a potential that we lose during our conditional experiencing in childhood? Are we discovering something new, or rediscovering something that was lost?

In the context of this volume, we need to consider a holistic approach, with both the drinking behaviour and psychological processes interrelating (as they do) within the therapeutic process. Each will contribute to, and inform, the other process, with a kind of feedback loop being generated, and the system evolving and developing by feeding off the changes made and the experiences that those changes bring into awareness. The more satisfying the experience of change is to the person, the greater their motivation to pursue change further. In the context of the topic of this volume, this process of psychological change, the rebalancing and integrating process, then becomes evidenced through a reduced need to binge drink to feel good, to feel normal, to feel a sense of belonging to a peer group.

Supervision

The supervision sessions are included in this volume to offer the reader insight into the nature of therapeutic supervision in the context of the counselling profession, a method of supervising that I term 'collaborative review'. For many trainee counsellors, the use of supervision can be something of a mystery, and it is hoped that this book will go a long way to unravelling this. In the supervision sessions,

I seek to demonstrate the application of the supervisory relationship. My intention is to show how supervision of the counsellor is very much a part of the process of enabling a client to work through issues, and in the context of this volume, issues associated with their binge drinking.

Many professions do not recognise the need for some form of personal and process supervision, and often what is offered is line management. However, counsellors are required to receive regular supervision in order to explore the dynamics of the relationship with the client, the impact of the work on the counsellor and on the client, to receive support, to encourage professional development of the counsellor and to provide an opportunity for an experienced co-professional to monitor the supervisee's work in relation to ethical standards and codes of practice. The supervision sessions are included because they are an integral part of the therapeutic process. It is also hoped that they will help readers from other professions to recognise the value of some form of supportive and collaborative supervision in order to help them become more authentically present with their own clients.

Merry describes what he termed 'collaborative inquiry' as a 'form of research or inquiry in which two people (the supervisor and the counsellor) collaborate or co-operate in an effort to understand what is going on within the counselling relationship and within the counsellor'. He emphasises how this 'moves the emphasis away from "doing things right or wrong" (which seems to be the case in some approaches to supervision) to "how is the counsellor being, and how is that way of being contributing to the development of the counselling relationship based on the core conditions"' (Merry, 2002, p. 173). Elsewhere, Merry describes the relationship between person-centred supervision and congruence, indicating that 'a state of congruence . . . is the necessary condition for the therapist to experience empathic understanding and unconditional positive regard' (Merry, 2001, p. 183). Effective person-centred supervision provides a means through which congruence can be promoted within the therapist. An overview of all of this is succinctly made by Merry: 'person-centred supervision is concerned with how you, the counsellor, form relationships with your clients, and how you can deepen your empathic understanding of them whilst remaining as congruent as you can and experiencing unconditional positive regard towards them', and adds that this places the onus on the therapist to be as open and non-defensive as they can be when discussing the way they think and feel about themselves in relationship with their clients (Merry, 2002, p. 170).

Tudor and Worrall (2004) have drawn together a number of theoretical and experiential strands from within and outside the person-centred tradition, in order to develop a theoretical position on the person-centred approach to supervision. In my view, this is a timely publication, defining the necessary factors for effective supervision within this way of working, and the respective responsibilities of both supervisor and supervisee in keeping with person-centred values and principles. They contrast person-centred working with other approaches to supervision, and emphasise the importance of the therapeutic space as a place within which practitioners 'can dialogue freely between their personal philosophy and the philosophical assumptions which underlie their chosen theoretical orientation' (Tudor and Worrall, 2004, 94–5). They affirm the values and attitudes of person-centred working, and explore their application to the supervisory relationship.

There are, of course, as many models of supervision as there are models of counselling. In this book the supervisor is seeking to apply the attitudinal qualities of the person-centred approach.

It is the norm for all professionals working in the healthcare and social care environment in this age of regulation to be formally accredited or registered, and to work to their own professional organisation's code of ethics or practice. For instance, counselling practitioners registered with the British Association for Counselling and Psychotherapy are required to have regular supervision and continuing professional development to maintain registration. While professions other than counsellors will gain much from this book in their work, it is essential that they follow the standards, safeguards and ethical codes of their own professional organisation, and are appropriately trained and supervised to work with them on the issues that arise. Also, in the context of the workplace, they should follow guidelines and policies specific to that particular organisation, with mindfulness of health and safety issues.

Dialogue format

The reader who has not read other titles in the *Living Therapy* series may find it takes a while to adjust to the dialogue format. Many of the responses offered by the counsellors, Rick and Sally, are reflections of what their respective clients, Gary and Carrie, have said. This is not to be read as conveying a simple repetition of the clients' words. Rather, the counsellors seek to voice empathic responses, often with a sense of 'checking out' that they are hearing accurately what the clients are saying. The client says something; the counsellor then conveys what they have heard, what they sense the client has sought to communicate to them, sometimes with the same words, sometimes with words that include a sense of what they feel is being communicated through the client's tone of voice, facial expression, or simply the relational atmosphere of the moment. The client is then enabled to confirm that they have been heard accurately, or correct the counsellor in their perception. The client may then explore more deeply what they have been saying or move on, in either case with a sense that they have been heard and warmly accepted. To draw this to the reader's attention, I have included some of the inner thoughts and feelings that are present within the individuals who form the narrative.

The sessions are a little compressed. It is also fair to say that clients will take different periods of time before choosing to disclose particular issues, and will also take varying lengths of time in working with their own process. This book is not intended to indicate in any way the length of time that may be needed to work with the kinds of issues that are being addressed. The counsellor needs to be open and flexible to the needs of the client. For some clients, the process would take a lot longer. But there are also clients who are ready to talk about difficult experiences almost immediately – sometimes not feeling that they have much choice in the matter, as their own organismic processes are already driving memories, feelings, thoughts and experiences to the surface and into daily awareness.

All characters in this book are fictitious and are not intended to bear resemblance to any particular person or persons. These fictional accounts are not aimed at trying to encompass all possible causes of binge drinking in young people; they simply highlight some of the behavioural, emotional, cognitive, psychological and social factors that can be associated with this increasing problem.

I am extremely encouraged by the increasing interest in the person-centred approach, the growing amount of material being published, and the realisation that relationship is a key factor in positive therapeutic outcome. There is currently much debate about theoretical developments within the person-centred world and its application. Discussions on the theme of Rogers' therapeutic conditions presented by various key members of the person-centred community have recently been published (Bozarth and Wilkins, 2001; Haugh and Merry, 2001; Wyatt, 2001; Wyatt and Sanders, 2002). Mearns and Thorne (2000) have produced a timely publication revising and developing key aspects of person-centred theory. Wilkins (2003) has produced a book that addresses most effectively many of the criticisms levelled against person-centred working (2003), and Embleton Tudor *et al* (2004) an introduction to the person-centred approach that places the theory and practice within a contemporary context. Mearns and Cooper (2005) have recently presented 'working at relational depth', Vincent (2005) draws together a rich mix of Rogers' references on the theme of *Being Empathic*, along with his own thinking in this area, and Levitt (2005) has edited a timely book exploring the theme of non-directivity. It seems there is an increasing stream of publications presenting and exploring the approach and its application in counselling and psychotherapy.

Recently, Howard Kirschenbaum (Carl Rogers' biographer) published an article entitled 'The current status of Carl Rogers and the person-centered approach'. In his research for this article he noted that from 1946 to 1986 there were 84 books, 64 chapters, and 456 journal articles published on Carl Rogers and the person-centred approach. In contrast, from 1987 to 2004 there were 141 books, 174 book chapters and 462 journal articles published. This is a clear trend towards more publications and, presumably, more readership and interest in the approach. Also, he noted that there were now some 50 person-centred publications available around the world, mostly journals, and there are now person-centred organisations in 18 countries, and 20 organisations overall. He also draws attention to the large body of research demonstrating the effectiveness of person-centred therapy, concluding that the person-centred approach is 'alive and well' and 'appears to be experiencing something of a revival, both in professional activity and academic respectability' (Kirschenbaum, 2005).

This is obviously a very brief introduction to the approach. Person-centred theory continues to develop as practitioners and theoreticians consider its application in various fields of therapeutic work and extend our theoretical understanding of developmental and therapeutic processes. At times it feels as if it has become more than just individuals; rather, it feels like a group of colleagues, based around the world, working together to penetrate deeper towards a more complete theory of the human condition, and this includes people from the many traditions and schools of thought. Person-centred or client-centred theory and practice has a key role in this process. Theories are being revisited and developed, new ideas speculated upon and new media explored for presenting the core values and philosophy of the person-centred approach. It is an exciting time.

PART I

Gary's story

'So, after a few beers in that environment, you begin to feel kind of different in some way?'

Gary nodded. 'Yeah, it's like, I don't know, different, yeah.'

'Different, and it's kind of hard to sort of describe what that "different" is like, yeah?'

Gary had lifted his arms by his sides, his fists clenched slightly.

Rick reflected his arm and hand movements. It felt to him like the kind of movement you might make before punching someone. He wondered how much the body movements were capturing the flavour of what the 'difference' was.

CHAPTER 1

Friday evening

Gary was getting himself dressed, looking forward to the evening (and weekend) ahead of him. Friday night, and he was going to have some fun. Get pissed, definitely, go clubbing, definitely, have a good time, for sure. Yeah, he was looking forward to enjoying himself. He worked hard and he liked his weekends, they were what he worked for. Have a good time, get out of his head, maybe a few pills, he didn't always do that, but sometimes, yeah, kept him going and made him feel good. He'd already spent a good half an hour, maybe a little more, getting himself ready. Well, that's what he liked to do. You had to look the part, yeah, and he was a man on a mission. He was going to pull, he didn't care who she was, he wasn't interested in any idea of a regular girlfriend. He had another look in the mirror. Yeah, he looked good. He was going to get really pissed and if anyone upset him, well, he wasn't looking for trouble, but if they started it, he'd sort it and tough shit on them. He didn't go out looking for trouble, but it happened sometimes, and he dealt with it. It was Friday night and, yeah, he lived for Friday night, and Saturday night, and, well, any other night if he went out with his mates.

He was planning a trip into town with Mal and Luke. They'd been mates for a while now. Known each other since school. Now they were all 18 and up for anything. Been on a couple of holidays together overseas as well. Yeah, had a lot of good times, and a lot of good shags as well. He was up for it, up for anything, especially after a few drinks. Been that way for a few years, particularly since leaving school.

The phone rang. It was Luke. 'You ready yet?'

'Nearly. You spoken to Mal?'

'Yeah, he's here. We'll be over in about 20 minutes.'

'OK, see you.' Gary hung up the phone and returned to the mirror, bit more time to just be sure he was looking his best. Made him feel good. He didn't know why, but he often felt like he wasn't at ease with himself, on edge, but he would push it aside. He knew he'd had a crap time in childhood, but he didn't think too much about that now.

Time passed, and it was soon approaching the time when Mal and Luke were due to arrive. They were planning to head down to the station – he only lived a five minute walk away. He looked around his room, at the posters on the walls, and the tumble of clothes on the chair. It was still light outside but he knew by the time they got into town it would be getting dark. The bar they went to was fairly near the station, and then they'd go on to a club that was only a few minutes' walk away as well. It was good, the bars and clubs so close to the station like that. Everyone went there. OK, yeah, could get a bit crazy later sometimes, but, well, you looked after yourself, get in first, that was his motto. Someone looks at you, go and sort it. Always made him feel good.

He sat down on the bed to tie up his shoes. Yeah, he felt good, he was going to have a good time. He stood up, and walked over to the window, he could see Mal and Luke heading towards his parents' house. He had another quick look in the mirror as he walked past, checked he'd got everything in his pocket, plenty of dosh and his card, and headed out the bedroom door and down the stairs. 'Mum, I'm out. Be back later. Don't wait up.' Not that you ever do, he thought to himself.

'You take care, don't go getting into any trouble, and get a taxi back if you're late.'

'Yeah, OK, I'll be fine.' The doorbell rang. 'That'll be Mal and Luke. Gotta go. Bye.'

'Bye.'

Gary opened the door. 'OK?'

'Yeah, course I am. So, come on, let's go and enjoy ourselves. I've been needing this all week. My boss has been a real pain in the arse. Fuck him!'

'Any arse in particular?' They all sniggered as they headed towards the railway station.

Counselling session 1: 'I don't have a problem with my drinking'

Monday 7 April

Gary walked across the car park at the doctor's surgery, thoughtlessly kicking a stone that was in his path. He heard it rattle off the hub cap of the green Fiat to his left. It made a nice sound. He didn't give it much more thought, he was more concerned with what the hell he was doing going to see a counsellor. It hadn't been his idea and he didn't see any point. Why did he need to talk to someone? What had he got to talk about? Just because the doctor thought he had a problem. Well, he didn't. Yeah, so he got into trouble sometimes, but that was no trouble, not really. Just how it was. Not a problem. He sorted his problems out, and this wasn't a problem. Waste of time, but the doctor had been insistent. So here he was, Monday morning, nine o'clock, to see some shrink about a problem he didn't have. Bloody marvellous.

He went into the surgery and stood in the queue at the reception desk. He didn't like queues, never liked waiting. He stood, hands in his pockets, staring at the back of the woman in front of him, wishing she wasn't there, in his way. Still, he then thought, if it makes the doctor happy, might get him off his back.

> In this instance the client has been referred for counselling for his binge drinking by his general practitioner (GP). There may not always be positive responses from the young person to such a referral, but some will engage in treatment via this route. It often depends on the way it is presented by the GP, and the relationship the young person has with their GP. It may also depend upon where the counsellor is located. My own experience of working in a GP surgery was that it offered scope for young people who were already familiar with the environment to attend. That seemed to help.

Eventually he got to the desk. The receptionist took his name and told him to wait and she'd call the counsellor to let him know that he had arrived. Gary went and sat down. He stared across the waiting area. What was he doing there? What was the doctor thinking about, telling him he had a problem with his drinking and he needed to talk to someone? He didn't have a problem, he didn't drink more than anyone else, and so what if he did get in fights, why was that a problem? Maybe for the other guy, he grinned at the thought of his last fight. Yeah, he'd sorted him out. So, he'd ended up in accident and emergency (A&E), but so what. It'd been worth it. What was the problem? He sat with his thoughts, feeling increasingly pissed off with being there and wondering how long the counsellor was going to be. He'd only been waiting two minutes.

'Hi, Gary?' He heard his name and looked up. A guy was looking his way.

'Yeah, that's me.'

'Hi, I'm Rick, the doctor asked you to see me?'

'Yeah.'

'OK, so, follow me, the room's along here.'

Gary followed Rick along the corridor, past the leaflet display and assorted posters warning of the dire consequences of various diseases. It wasn't how he wanted to spend his Monday morning. He followed Rick into a room on the right.

'Take a seat, whichever.'

Rick went to the seat nearest to him, which happened to be closest to the door.

'So, Doctor James has referred you, and I assume he gave you the information leaflet about the counselling service, what we offer, how it's confidential and what that means?'

Gary was looking out the window. 'Yeah, yeah, he did.'

'Any questions, anything you weren't clear about?'

'Nah.'

Rick nodded, very aware of the tension that was present in the room. His instant sense was that Gary didn't want to be there. Not all his clients did, and certainly not everyone who was referred to him with an alcohol problem. Although he was a general counsellor, the surgery knew of his experience of working with people with alcohol problems, so they tended to refer people to him.

'OK, so, what I know from the referral letter is that you'd been in a fight recently, alcohol related, and the doctor felt you might benefit from seeing me. Whether that's your view, I don't know. But I'm happy to listen and give you some time and you can decide whether it's helpful, whether you want to continue coming, it's up to you.'

Gary was still looking out of the window. He snorted. He didn't want to say much. He didn't have a problem. It was the doctor who had the problem. He shook his head as he thought about it, still looking out of the window. He didn't say anything.

'You don't want to be here, do you?'

The counsellor is being transparent in what he senses to be the situation and experience for his client. It's not that the client has directly said this, but his manner, his demeanour, is communicating this to the counsellor. It can be a powerful response, it brings reality into the room, into the relationship, into what is passing between client and counsellor. It is not voiced as a judgement, a criticism. It is an attitude that the counsellor will accept. The person-centred approach requires that the counsellor accepts how the client feels, warmly and unconditionally, and that they do not bring into the relationship an intent to seek to change the client in any specific way. The client is there, he doesn't want to be, the counsellor senses this to be the client's reality, and he voices it in an accepting manner.

No. I don't see why I have to be. I haven't got a problem.' He shrugged, still looking out of the window.

'Mhmm, no problems, everything's fine, yeah?'

'Nothing I can't sort out.'

'Yep, you've got it all under control, yeah?'

'I mean, what's . . .' He shook his head again. He turned to look at Rick, who was looking his way, and looked him in the eyes. 'I mean, why do I have to see you, no disrespect, but, I mean, I don't know. He thinks I'd find it helpful to talk to you.' He shook his head. 'I told him, "I'm OK, I don't have a problem". But he didn't take much notice, told me I should see you, said you'd be able to, I don't know, give me time to talk about things. But what have I got to talk about? I haven't got a problem.'

'OK, so it's like he thinks you have a problem, but you don't, he thinks it would be helpful for you to come and talk to me, and you're wondering what the hell you're doing here.' Rick was intentionally direct in his response, seeking to be upfront. His experience told him that this was the best way to be. Say it as it was, or as he was experiencing it. Don't get into 'counsellor-speak', just level with the client. At least that way the relationship could begin to be established and that, as far as Rick was concerned, was what really mattered. He accepted, more than accepted, he knew that to the degree that he could form a relationship, and for that relationship to develop therapeutically, then there would be the possibility for something constructive to occur for the client. He accepted Rogers' 'necessary and sufficient conditions for constructive personality change', and his role was to offer the therapeutic qualities as a contribution to ensuring those conditions were present in the room, in the relationship. He had deliberately spoken not loudly, but not quietly, again seeking to convey a sense of his presence. He sought to match the tone in his client's voice.

'Yeah, yeah, you've got it. That's how it is.' Gary nodded. Yeah, at least this guy seemed to hear how it was. Pity his GP hadn't heard him like that, he probably wouldn't have had to be here now, wasting his time.

Note that the counsellor has not launched into a formal assessment. The focus is being placed on establishing contact and relationship with the client, on offering the therapeutic conditions. From a person-centred perspective, therapy starts where there is contact. To formally assess will bring a directive element into the therapeutic process, setting a tone for the relationship that will be built. The client will then experience the counsellor as someone who probes, asking questions about areas of his life and awareness that the client may not want or feel ready to disclose. The person-centred therapist will be wanting to let the client communicate what they want to disclose, when they want to. So, the emphasis is on listening, on communicating empathy and warm acceptance, on being non-directive, and on letting the client communicate whatever it is that they wish the counsellor to hear. This is a significant difference between person-centred therapy and most other forms of counselling.

There are, of course, settings in which there is a requirement for an assessment, for a history. Where this is the case, then it should either be undertaken by someone else other than the therapist, or it should be made clear by the therapist that some basic information is required by the agency. The person-centred counsellor will not want to invade the client's inner (and outer) world. The best way is for information to build up over time. Many clients don't immediately want to tell you their family history, it may contain experiences they are uncomfortable with, or do not wish to share with someone they have only just met. Why should they? The person-centred therapist is more concerned with communicating to the client that they, the client, have the power to choose what they wish to say, and when they want to say it. This is fundamental, setting an important tone for the building of the therapeutic relationship.

'OK, and he was saying he thought you specifically had a problem with your drinking, and that's what you're pretty clear you don't have.'

'Mhmm, and that's what's important, yeah, feeling, yeah, you can handle it.'

'Yeah, your drinking isn't causing you a problem.'

'Nah.' He pulled face. No, it wasn't a problem, it was how it was. He didn't have a
  problem. So what the hell was he doing there? Why didn't people let him be?
  At least this guy, Rick, wasn't pushing him. In fact, Rick seemed to quite accept
  what he was saying. That was actually a bit of a relief, not that he would have
  agreed with anyone who said he'd got a problem. The doctor had pissed him off
  insisting that he came and saw this guy. Oh well, time was passing, he wouldn't
  have to hang around for too long now.
'Ok, so, the fight, the hospital, that's kind of OK.'
'It happens.'
'Sounds like an occupational hazard.' Rick spoke how he felt.
Gary shrugged. 'S'pose it is. Well, I mean, you know, it happens, Friday night,
  you're out there, get tanked up, someone gets in your way so you sort it, you
  know?'
'Happens a lot, you mean?'
'Yeah, yeah, it does, it's how it is. I mean, you know, bevvied up and, well, yeah,
  something usually happens and, well, yeah, I like to get stuck in, you know?'
'Mhmm, something goes off and you're, what, part of it, and you like to get
  stuck in.'
'Sometimes, depends. Sometimes it's someone says something, looks at you, you
  know, gets in your space. Or knocks your drinks. Fuck, I hate that. Some bastards can't bloody well look where they're going and, well, yeah, I react.'
'So, someone does something, like knock your drink over or cause you to spill it
  and you react, yeah?' Rick kept his tone of voice accepting towards what Gary
  was saying. He wanted to keep it light, keep it conversational, keep ensuring
  that Gary felt heard, that his attitude, his view on drinking and getting into
  fights was being heard and accepted.

This is important. It's not that the counsellor agrees with Gary's behaviour – the counsellor isn't there to pass judgement. But he is there to
accept what the client is communicating, accept the way that the client
sees themselves and their behaviour. Of course, the client might interpret
the counsellor's listening and acceptance as being an agreement with how
he chooses to behave. But what is crucial is the counsellor's intention. Gary
likes to drink and get into fights, and he does not see it as a problem. Rick
accepts that this is Gary's experience and he does not judge Gary on this.
The person-centred counsellor will accept how the client needs to be,
accept the content of their inner (and outer) world. They may experience
personal reactions to something that the client says, we all do, we are
human beings, as counsellors we are in contact and relationship with our
clients, but the person-centred counsellor will be focusing on maintaining
empathy and unconditional positive regard towards their client, and on
communicating these in a manner such that the client is able to perceive
them as being present.

'Yeah, too right. Bastards.'

'Mhmm, bastards for being so clumsy, yeah?'

'Yeah.' Gary hadn't really thought about it but he was becoming more animated as he spoke, he was becoming more in touch with his feelings. 'You know, you dress up, take a bit of trouble and, well, I just don't accept it. And, yeah, I'll want to sort it, you know?'

'Yeah, and by sort it you mean . . . ?'

'Give 'em a bit of the verbal, maybe, tell 'em what I think of them, yeah?'

'So you give them the verbal, tell them what you think about them.'

'Yeah, and, well, if they react then I'll have a go. I don't give a shit then. I'll go for them.' Gary felt himself smile – yeah, made him feel good. He didn't know why, didn't even think about it like that, had no reason to, he just knew it was all part of the buzz.

'Mhmm, and that can happen, what, at any time when you're out?'

> The counsellor has strayed away from a non-directive stance. He has asked a question in order to gain information. He is moving the client away from what he is specifically communicating. A more person-centred response would have been to have said something along the lines of: 'Mhmm, they react, you're at the stage of not giving a shit and you go for them'. The client is then much more likely to feel heard. What the counsellor has actually said does not communicate to the client that they have been heard, only that the counsellor is concerned with wanting to know how often it happens. This is the counsellor's agenda from within his frame of reference, and is not a person-centred response.

'Well, yeah, I guess, usually later in the evening.' Rick felt suddenly hesitant.

'OK, so as the evening goes by you're more likely to react and have a go, yeah?'

'Yeah, yeah, I s'pose I do. Hadn't really thought about it like that but, yeah, well, I mean, that's how it is. Idiots who can't take their booze, you know, stumbling idiots. Yeah, they deserve a whackin', you know? Ought to stay at home if they can't take it.'

> A client responding along the lines of 'I hadn't really thought about it like that' is a clear indication that the counsellor has introduced something from their frame of reference into the client's experience. Gary's hesitancy is a reaction to what Rick has said. His flow of experiencing and communication has been disturbed by the counsellor. It may not just be what Rick has said, but also the way he has said it. Why does it matter how often? What does asking this communicate to the client? It could be felt to be judgemental.

'Mhmm, so by that time of the evening you're up for it, anyone who gets in your space, looks at you too long, causes you to spill your drink, and you'll have a go? It's what they deserve.'

Gary nodded. Yeah, it was. He felt quite hot suddenly. Yeah, this guy did understand what it was like. Wasn't what he expected. Counsellor, well, you think of
someone . . . , he wasn't sure, some kind of shrink who'd get in your head and
mess you about, tell you you'd had a crap childhood, blame it all on that. No, he
had no time for that. Yeah, OK, so he had had a crap childhood, but what of it?
Most of the kids from his way had. Broken homes, gangs, you had to get respect
to survive. But it wasn't really crap, you got by. You did what you had to do,
that was how it was. Yeah, he'd had trouble, few run-ins with the law. Just
having a good time, a few laughs. Do what you had to do. That was how it
was. They'd told him last time it would be prison if it happened again. Well, he
didn't want that, he wasn't a criminal. He'd got his job and didn't want to
lose that. He, yeah, he didn't like the idea of that. But he put the concern
aside. Didn't do you any good worrying about things like that. What mattered
was that he had respect from his mates, from the people that mattered to him,
and anyone else that crossed him. At least, he felt he had respect and that was
what was important, really important. Made him feel good. Made him feel alive,
normal, yeah, you had to have respect and, well, being up for a fight when you
needed to, yeah, that gave you respect. And drinking, that gave you respect
too. Getting pissed. Shagging any girl who gave you a second look as well.
He felt himself smiling as he thought of some of the good times he'd had.

Rick was obviously aware of Gary lapsing into silence. He didn't know quite
what he was thinking about but he had noticed him smile. Well, he thought
to himself, here's someone with some pretty clear ideas about what a good
night's all about, he's really into the violence around his drinking. Was he
simply violent, angry, for whatever reason, all the time, or did the alcohol
draw it out, open him up to it? He thought of the image he'd read about,
how alcohol can, for some people, seemingly numb their emotions, but for
other people it opens them up.

> 'My experience of working with clients who have alcohol problems suggests
> that a large part of their difficulty lies with their sensitivity to their emotions.
> For some this is a cause of alcohol use, but it can also be an effect of excessive
> alcohol intake as well. For some people alcohol can shut away the emotions;
> for others it opens them up, as though there is a trap-door to the feeling
> nature. Alcohol oils the hinge, leaving some people experiencing it swinging
> shut while for others it swings wide open' (Bryant-Jefferies, 2001, p. 218).

He knew that for a lot of people alcohol took them to a place in themselves where
they encountered feelings that they could not control. But, well, it was speculation as far as Gary was concerned. His task was to build a relationship with
Gary, try and get alongside him, convey a sense of the inner and outer world
that Gary was describing and experiencing. And trust the therapeutic process.
He respected Gary's silence, at least he was outwardly silent; whether his inner
world was silent was another matter.

'So, you think I've got a problem?' Gary had decided to ask the question, feeling sure that Rick would say no, and then he could put an end to this counselling stuff and head off to work. Well, actually, he wasn't in a hurry to go to work, but then, well, he could take his time getting in.

'Depends on how we define a problem. Seems to me that what you've described, getting into fights and ending up at the hospital to get patched up, for you, that doesn't feel like a problem.'

'Yeah, it's what happens.'

'Mhmm. And so I respect that as being how you experience it.'

Gary felt suspicious. The way Rick was speaking sounded different. 'So, what are you saying?'

'I guess I'm saying that if I experienced that I'd feel it was a problem. But that's me. For you, it's not a problem, it's what happens and you get on with it.'

Gary still felt uneasy. What was this guy saying, then, that he thought he did have a problem. 'It's what happens. Yeah, maybe, yeah, maybe I do . . . , yeah, but it's not a problem.' Gary felt like he'd had enough. He wanted to go.

'Yeah, and I hear you, Gary. It's what happens and you're OK about it, and it really isn't a problem.'

'Well, I mean, how would you describe a drinking problem?'

'How would I describe a drinking problem?'

'Yeah. I don't have a problem with it but you say you'd think it was a problem if it happened to you.' Rick was aware that the atmosphere in the room had changed, he could feel an edge to it. Well, was it the atmosphere – what did that mean? Maybe it was simply that he felt different, that he had tightened up inside. Hmm. But he was clear that he had to try and keep his perception separate from his client's, and to focus on the client's view, and he had slid away from that. And yet he was simply saying it as he saw it. Then again, that response he'd just made, 'and I hear you', who was he trying to convince? Himself, or Gary who he could well appreciate was probably not feeling heard? Yes, he realised he hadn't been authentic in saying that he respected Gary's view. He didn't agree with it, it wasn't his view, and that had disrupted his empathy and unconditional positive regard. He'd broken the therapeutic alliance.

Content, material, experiences within the counsellor can so easily intrude into the therapeutic process, hence the importance of self-discipline and self-awareness in the counsellor. The fact that Rick sees things differently from Gary has affected what he has said, and very likely his tone of voice and probably his facial expression. The client will feel uneasy, sensing that his counsellor is not being real with him, and therefore what is then said becomes untrustworthy. It can be obvious and it can be subtle, and the person-centred counsellor has to guard against this and be open to reflect on the possibility that their own thoughts, ideas and feelings are affecting their responding to their client in a way that disrupts the therapeutic alliance.

'For me drinking is a problem when it causes problems. It's then a case of deciding whether what you experience when you're out drinking is causing you a problem, or not, or anyone else.' Rick had realised that, given what had just happened, his being congruent and transparent was now more important than ever.

For some reason Gary heard Mal's voice in his head, telling him to back off, telling him that he knew what he was like, give the other guy a chance, it was an accident. But that was Mal, he didn't react the same. Yeah, it was usually Mal pulling him away, telling him to 'calm down, for fuck's sake'.

'I don't think it's a problem.' Rick noticed a slight change in Gary's voice, slightly more reflective, less heated. He altered his own tone of voice to convey his empathy and responsiveness to what Gary was saying and the way he was saying it.

'Mhmm, so, OK, you don't think your drinking causes you problems.' He spoke slowly giving Gary time to hear what he was saying.

'Well, no, I mean, you know, it would be good to maybe have a night when there isn't any trouble. But, well, it doesn't happen, does it? It's what goes off after a few beers.'

'So, what you're saying is that while it feels like it might be good to have a night without trouble, in reality it's not something that happens once people have had a few beers. It's certainly not your experience.'

'No. No. But, yeah, well, maybe it might be good sometimes to get home and not, well, not be nursing a few bruises, but the other guy always comes off worse.' Mostly, he thought, but his pride wasn't going to let him say anything about, yeah, well, that one guy'd been maybe a bit too big to take on. Not that he thought that at the time. It was a few weeks back, this guy'd knocked into him in the bar as he went out. Gary'd gone after him, given him some verbal and, well, yeah OK, he'd had to have a couple of stitches and had lost a tooth. Yeah, sometimes it felt like, well, yeah, sometimes he had allowed himself to wonder about it all, usually the next day when he was feeling a bit battered and hung over. And sometimes he couldn't remember what had happened, like he'd blanked it all out. That was weird. Still, maybe sometimes it was best not to know.

Alcohol blackout is not passing out, but memory loss. A person lives a period of their lives and say they wake up one morning with no awareness of what they did the previous day. They have been up and about, but the way they process experience and store memory is impaired. It can be quite common among heavy drinkers, and is definitely an indication of alcohol damage. It can cause other problems, for instance, agoraphobia as the person begins to fear going out because they do not know what they have been doing, who they might have upset, who they might need to avoid. And as one client said to me, 'once people realise I've been in blackout they start telling me I borrowed money from them. What do I do? I don't know if they're right or not'.

'So, sometimes, not all of the time, but sometimes you find yourself wishing it could have been different, yeah?'

'Yeah, sometimes. You get tired of it, you know.'

'Mhmm, sort of wears you down, do you mean?'

'Yeah, sometimes, you know, it would be good to just have a few pints without the grief. Yeah, sometimes it would be good to just go out, have a few pints, a few laughs, you know, and not get the hassle.'

'Yeah few pints, no grief, no hassle, just a few laughs and back home.'

'Sometimes. And then well, you don't think like that, do you, I mean, not after the first couple.'

'You find you're thinking differently after a couple of beers, do you mean?'

'Yeah, well . . .' Gary felt unsure and uneasy. What was he saying? 'Yeah, different, but that's not a problem.'

'No, feeling different like that doesn't give you a problem.'

'No.' Gary hesitated. 'No, no it doesn't.'

'No, finding that, what, after a couple of pints or so you're feeling different, maybe not so bothered about there not being any hassle.'

'I'm probably looking for it.' Gary hadn't planned to say it but the words came out. He tightened his lips. Fuck's sake, what was he saying?

Here we see the emergence of material denied to the client's awareness. This isn't something he has really thought about himself. He doesn't see himself as someone who looks for trouble, at least, not when he's in a non-alcohol-affected state of mind. When he's alcohol affected, this changes. Arguments happen and Gary sorts it out, as he sees it, and in the only way he knows when he is in that frame of reference. It is likely that alcohol disinhibits Gary to the degree that whatever internal mechanism exists within him to contain his aggression breaks down. It is probably that his need to not be like his father is contributing to this, his earlier experiences of what violence can do, and how it left him feeling. But, alcohol in the system takes away this self-control, the need to not be aggressive breaks down under pressure from the need to feel powerful in the situation that has arisen. He's not going to let himself feel bullied or powerless.

'OK, and let's just be clear, after a couple of pints or so you're looking for hassle, yeah, looking for trouble?'

'Well, yeah, I guess so, sort of.' This didn't feel at all comfortable suddenly. And he didn't like feeling like that. 'What're you saying?'

'I'm trying to be clear about what you're telling me and checking out that what I'm hearing is what you're saying.'

'Hmm.' Gary went into silence and looked out of the window. He wanted to talk about something else. This guy was beginning to irritate him. And yet, somehow, he did seem to sort of understand in some kind of way that he couldn't really make sense of. Like he did listen. Not that he really wanted to be listened

to, but he wasn't someone who just sounded off, telling him how he'd got a problem. And yet . . . , it sort of felt that somehow he was, at least, if not telling him,
sort of, well, sort of . . . , yeah. He looked over to Rick, looking into his eyes.

Rick returned the eye contact. He felt quite accepting of Gary now, of what he was
telling him. Yes, he could well appreciate that for Gary none of it was a problem. He was well used to going out, getting tanked up, getting into a state of
mind where he reacted, got into fights, maybe regretted it the next day, felt different when he wasn't alcohol affected, and then, well, a few more drinks and
the cycle would be set off again. Somehow recognising this was helping Rick to
feel that warm acceptance for his client. And it enabled him to hold the eye contact with a greater degree of assurance.

Gary respected the fact that Rick was returning his gaze and he looked somehow . . . , the word that came to mind was 'solid'. He snorted and looked away.
'So, what now?'

'What do you want to do now?'

Gary was biting his lip. 'I don't know. I'm not some alcy, you know, those guys
down by the river, always fucking pissed.'

The client has made a connection and a sudden jump, or so it can appear
from outside his frame of reference. For the client, however, he is simply
expressing connections that he has within his own thought processes. The
client has a need to say what he has said – it is important for him to distinguish himself from the people he is referring to as 'alcys'. Such a comment
might be made in a very derogatory way, and this could be a challenge to the
counsellor, who may feel very different. From my own experience, I find it
hard to warmly accept such views, having experienced therapeutic relationship with dependent drinkers and gained insight into the often tragic and
traumatic life experiences that have contributed to their drinking choices.
However, the counsellor has to be able to empathise with the inner world
of the client, with their perception, their reality.

Rick appreciated the extreme that Gary was comparing himself with. He thought
he could recall a statistic that the classic down-and-out drinker represented
only a few per cent of people with alcohol problems. But he wasn't there to
exchange statistics. Gary was making a comparison that he knew would
mean he could see himself as not having an alcohol problem. Lots of people
did that. Of course, the people that he was referring to, the local street drinkers,
many of them may have started out like Gary, but he wasn't there to try and
persuade him of this. His role was clear: listen to his client, warmly accept him
as the person that he is and let him know he is being heard. Get into relationship – therapeutic relationship – with him and what would follow, emerge,
well, that couldn't be second guessed. What would happen, would happen.

Rick suppressed a smile; yeah, what happens, happens, and he could suddenly
appreciate the similarity and difference with what Gary had said about how

trouble, fights happened when people had a few beers. Yeah, put people in that relational environment and you get a set of experiences and behaviours, same as you did when you put someone in a therapeutic experience. It was just that generally the behaviours and experiences were somewhat different, though not always. Both could contribute to the emergence, expression and release of emotion. So many people preferred a few beers to talking, or needed a few beers in order to talk, but by then the alcohol had caused them to connect with another part of themselves that would bring with it a set of thoughts, feelings and behaviours that, well, that could then be problematic to the person, or to other people.

Rick responded to Gary's comment. 'Not like the guys down by the river, not always pissed.'

'I can control it, that's the difference.' Gary had looked up and was staring at Rick with a certain attitude, Rick couldn't quite define it, but it seemed like there was an element of menace, and then it was gone. It was momentarily unsettling. As if he had seen a glimpse of some part of Gary, and then it wasn't there. He noted it to himself and acknowledged to himself that it had felt different, that he had felt different. Did he feel threatened? No, not exactly, although it did leave him with a sense that Gary could lose it. Just a brief glimpse and yet . . . It seemed to somehow convey so much. But it was still only a part of Gary and, of course, it was his own interpretation of his experience, he could be wrong. He didn't think he was and it was good to acknowledge to himself the reality of the experience. But he had to respond to Gary, to what he had just said.

'That's what makes the difference, knowing that you can control your drinking.' Rick spoke directly with a certain deliberation, wanting to communicate in quite a matter-of-fact way what Gary had said. This was important. He recognised how therapeutically important it was for Gary to feel that what he was saying, how he saw things, was heard. Yes, the temptation could be to allow the response to be affected by thinking and feeling differently, and yes, he knew that had happened earlier in the session. But he felt more focused now.

Gary nodded. It wasn't the alcohol that was a problem. He knew his limit. Yeah, he knew he drank heavily, but that was his choice. He was in control of his drinking. 'Yeah.'

Rick nodded. He didn't see any need to say anything more. It seemed that Gary had heard his empathic response. Gary was affirming his sense of being in control of his drinking and he wasn't going to disturb this. His role was to convey his empathy and acceptance of Gary's inner world.

Gary didn't feel like saying anything else, didn't see much point. He felt he'd said what he wanted to say, made himself clear. No need to say anything else. He didn't have a problem, it was a waste of time being here and he'd had enough. He continued to sit, turning his head away and rubbing the back of his neck. He felt stiff. Needed a few beers, that would set him right. Yeah, he'd make a point of sinking a few that night, yeah, maybe prove something to himself. He was no alcy, just liked a few beers, normal, what everyone else did, get a few down himself, have a few laughs, maybe pull, yeah, good times, fucking good times. He was staring down at the carpet.

Rick, meanwhile, felt the shift in atmosphere. His sense was that there was now once again a real sense of distance between himself and Gary. It felt to him that he hadn't distanced himself, he felt he was still attentive. Had Gary pulled back, withdrawn? It felt like that but he didn't want to get into some way of thinking that wanted to blame. Things were as they were. Counselling wasn't an every-day experience. Maybe Gary contrasting himself with the guys he called 'alcys' was unsettling, or maybe it had caused Gary to experience an affirmation that he didn't have a problem. Like he said, he felt he had control of his drinking. It was the behaviour that followed, but that was a different story. Anyway, Gary needed to be how he needed to be now, in the session, and it was OK.

'So, we've only a few more minutes, I guess it's been an unusual experience being here?'

'Bit weird but, yeah, OK, but I haven't got a problem, I control my drinking, yeah?'

'Mhmm. Doesn't cause you a problem, you have it under control.'

Gary shook his head. 'Nah, stuff we were talking about, fighting and stuff, that's well, that's how it is, not a problem. Bit of a laugh, you know?' He stuck his jaw out as he finished speaking.

'Bit of a laugh, that's how it feels, I mean, really feels?'

'Yeah, well, you know. I mean, yeah, you get pumped up, someone gives you a bit of lip, gives you a look and, well, yeah, you get in there, you know? Jungle out there, you've got to survive.'

'Mhmm, and that's what you do, survive?'

Gary nodded. And he was aware as well of that feeling inside himself that also sort of wanted a bit of quiet as well sometimes. But he pushed that aside. He didn't really understand it anyway. No, get tanked up, few laughs, mess around, and if someone got in the way, well, too bad for them. It pissed him off, he'd like a night out without hassle, but when it happened, yeah, he dealt with it.

The session drew to a close, but not before Gary had asked Rick whether he wanted to see him again.

'Do you want to come back, maybe in a couple of weeks and see how things are?'

Gary shrugged. He could manage that. He knew the GP'd probably have a go if he didn't, not that that particularly worried him. But he didn't need the hassle. Yeah, he could come back, something about it sort of appealed in some way, but he didn't really understand why. Didn't really think about it. Seemed like this guy wasn't telling him he had a problem, so he wasn't sure why he was there, but, well, yeah, he'd come back – well, he didn't want to get into some long discussion about it. Get out and worry about it in a couple of weeks. Maybe he'd come back, maybe he wouldn't.

The session ended with Rick telling Gary he'd drop a line to the GP to let him know that Gary had attended and that he was coming back in a couple of weeks.

'Yeah, sure, you gonna tell him I've got a problem?'

Rick smiled. 'I'll tell him you came today and that you don't experience your drinking as a problem.'

'Yeah, but that's not how you see it, is it?'

'No, I've got to be honest, I don't, but I respect that you do. That's how it is.'

'I'm not an alcy.'

'I'm not saying you are.'

'So what are you saying?'

'I don't think you have as much control as you think you have.'

'I can control my drinking.'

''Mhmm, and that's how you feel and that's how you experience it, under control, not causing any problems, what you do. Yeah?'

'Yeah.' He paused. 'Yeah.'

'OK, see you in a couple of weeks.'

Gary left, strangely unsettled by what had just been said, but he didn't know why. Yeah, he thought, 'course I've got it under control. Just get into a few fights, that's all, not a problem. I can handle it.' But as he walked away from the surgery he was thinking, sort of quiet inside, it felt strange, he felt strange, a little light-headed – and that was without a few drinks. He couldn't make sense of it, and gave up trying. No, he would be out with his mates later, but he wasn't going to tell them anything about the counselling. That'd piss 'em off for sure, or they'd have a good laugh about it. He wasn't sure that he wanted that, though he wasn't sure why. The guy'd got to him, got in his head. Just listening, weird. And he'd held eye contact. Sort of respected him for that. But thinking he'd got a problem? Well, he hadn't, and that was that, and he hadn't anything to prove to anyone. He speeded up his pace as he headed to work.

Rick had written his notes but was still reflecting on his experience of his encounter with Gary. He could see that there was something hidden, something angry, something that could lash out. He was sure that the alcohol and this part of Gary were linked in some way. Alcohol releasing pent-up anger? Perhaps. Or did he have his own demons that alcohol got him away from and he'd just lose it, maybe leave him a bit paranoid towards other people, more reactive, volatile? He could sit and speculate, but what mattered was what happened in the session, how well he could offer the therapeutic conditions and how they were received by Gary. He could only imagine what Gary made of counselling, having some guy like himself sitting listening, looking at him. Not normal, at least, not in a society that seems to discourage eye contact. But what of Gary? What would he make of it? He had no idea.

He hoped he'd come back. He couldn't make him, of course. He knew that wasn't the way, he had to trust that Gary would choose whatever was right for him. But what would feel right for him? Therapy, being listened to, could feel so wrong to people who were not used to it or if some part of themselves felt strongly threatened by it. Still, he seemed happy to accept another appointment, and only then would he know if Gary was up for another session of counselling.

Points for discussion

- Your reactions to the session? What do you feel towards Gary? Would these feelings be an obstacle to your offering him counselling?

- Evaluate Rick's empathic responding and warm acceptance of Gary. Do you feel they were sufficiently conveyed and received?
- There were times when Rick chose not to voice his inner thoughts and feelings. Congruence does not mean openly voicing whatever you think or feel. Discuss the role of congruence in the therapeutic process.
- The counsellor has not explored with the client exactly how much he is drinking. The focus has been client led, the emphasis was on Gary's perception of his drinking and why it isn't a problem – though he says it would be good to just have a few quiet beers sometimes. What are your thoughts on this?
- If you had felt threatened or unsafe in the session, what would you have done? How would you have matched your response to person-centred theory?
- What would you take to supervision from this session if you were the counsellor?

Write notes for this session.

CHAPTER 2

Later that night

The bar was busy. They had really been enjoying themselves. They'd had a few drinks at a bar in town and they were feeling good. Yes, Mal and Luke knew that Gary could get a bit out of control, but that's how he was. They sometimes felt he went a little over the top, but they were used to it.

They left the bar and headed round to the club nearby. It was hot inside, really hot, and they were glad they'd not overdressed. It wasn't long before they were dancing, though only after another couple of rounds of drinks at the bar. The music was fast and the beat incessant. They were used to it.

After a while Gary began to tire, he felt thirsty again and made his way to the bar. He noticed a guy with a girl, she seemed drop-dead gorgeous and deliberately knocked into him as he walked past. He kept looking at her.

The guy looked briefly and moved away, pushing her with him, but she looked back at Gary. He smiled and raised an eyebrow, and his glass. She smiled back. She'd only just met the guy she was with. There was something innocent in Gary's face, and yet strong, and she liked that.

'You better take care of her, mate, or I'll have her away from you.' He grinned as he turned away, and took a few gulps of his beer. He returned to the bar to where Mal and Luke were standing, both grinning.

'Did you see her?'

'Sure we did, fuck's sake, man, you really are up for it tonight.'

'Something to prove to myself, that's all.' Gary was thinking back to the counselling session. Think I've got a problem? No way, I can look after myself, I can handle it. He was nodding and smiling to himself.

It was about 20 minutes later and the girl that Gary had been eyeing up was heading towards him. 'Like to buy me a drink?'

'Yeah, sure, love to.' He moved away from Mal and Luke. 'What's your name?'

'Mandy.'

'I'm Gary. So, what'll you have.'

Mandy told him and Gary turned to order.

'What the fuck's your game?' Gary heard the voice and turned. It was matey from a few minutes back, not looking too happy.

Mandy put on such a sweet smile. 'I think he's buying me a drink.' She turned away. Gary felt himself being pushed from behind. That was all it took. Gary was ready, and he feared no one, not the way he was feeling just at that moment. He turned and pushed back, knocking the guy backwards, he came back at him but Gary was ready. Yeah, he'd had a few drinks, but he'd still got some co-ordination left, and lashed out, knocking him over. 'I'll fucking have you.' The guy was getting to his feet, and turned away. Gary was set to go after him but it was Mal who held him back. 'Come on, he's not worth it, let him go, you've got his girl. He's not worth it.'

Gary could feel the anger still inside himself. He didn't like being pushed around. He stood for a while staring in the direction the other guy had taken, then slowly shook his head and turned his attention to Mandy. 'Known him long?'

'No, picked him up earlier, glad you put him down, bit of a creep.'

By now a couple of large guys had come over – security.

'OK, we saw what happened, you're out.'

'What, fuck's sake, what's your problem?'

'We saw you lash out, we don't need you in here, Out!'

Gary wasn't having any of it and in his state of mind the size of the two security guys wasn't an issue. He took a swing at the one nearest him. He missed and was pinned against the bar. 'You're out, come on.' There was a slight pause, 'and you two, you're with him, you're out as well'. Gary was somewhat unceremoniously taken away, Mal and Luke followed, all were protesting. Mandy watched, she thought it was kind of funny, guys fighting over her. Yeah, she liked that. She followed along to see what was going to happen.

Outside the security men let Gary go, telling him in no uncertain terms to go home. Gary was still angry, he really was boiling. He wasn't going to let them get away with it and he rushed back at them, but one of the security guys got him round the neck and held him. Mal and Luke looked at each other and went for him, he loosened his grip and Gary got free. They dragged him away, 'come on, let's get away'. Gary was reluctant, he was still swearing and pointing at the security guys who stood, quite dispassionately; all in a night's work as far as they were concerned.

Mandy had seen the fight that had broken out and decided that she wasn't sure she wanted to follow them. She went back into the club.

Counselling session 2: client does not attend

Monday 21 April

Rick sat in the counselling room. Gary was due for his appointment. He wasn't sure whether Gary would attend. He hoped so, but he had a kind of gut feeling around it that left him with a sense of not feeling surprised if he didn't show. Reception had not called to let him know that Gary had arrived, but he decided to go out to check. Sometimes messages didn't always get relayed to him. He went out to the waiting area to see, but Gary wasn't there. Rick spoke briefly to the receptionist and then returned to the counselling room.

He sat and continued to try and maintain his own openness to whatever he was experiencing. He wanted to maintain himself in a prepared state should Gary arrive. After all, it was Gary's time and while, yes, it was frustrating sometimes when clients did not show up, nevertheless he wanted to be prepared in himself to receive Gary.

He found himself reflecting on the previous session and wondering how the world looked from Gary's perspective. He knew that he only had a limited sense of this and that he shouldn't make assumptions. He had worked with other young people and was aware how often there was a strong sense of living for the day, of not thinking too far into the future. That wasn't the case for everyone he had seen; occasionally he had had clients who were late teenagers who did have a sense of the future, who were trying to work towards creating some life for themselves that had a longer time frame, but that was the exception. He pondered about his own past. Was he that different? He hadn't really had much of an idea of what he had wanted to do with his life, he'd gone to university but with no strong sense of what he had wanted to do. It was only much later in his life, and after a career in the field of local government, that he had begun to take a strong interest in counselling. He'd been interested in working with young people for many years, and had been involved with local initiatives to give young people some interests and a place to go. It had been chatting to young people that had left him thinking about training in counselling and, well, one thing had led to another and now he was a counsellor himself.

He brought his thoughts back to Gary and to that last session. He, Rick, could see how the alcohol was a problem, and could see how, for Gary, it wasn't. And, in the final analysis, his role as a person-centred counsellor was to warmly accept Gary as he was, as he saw things, to gain and communicate an understanding of what Gary felt and thought, and how he chose to act in the world. He called reception on the phone. No sign of Gary. He decided to spend another five minutes waiting and, if he still did not arrive, make himself a cup of tea and decide what response to make.

Gary did not arrive and Rick drafted a letter, copying it to Dr James. He wanted to write the letter in such a way that he reached out to Gary. He always felt it was so important to make the letter personal. He hated those form letters that some agencies used. For Rick what was important was that the letter was, in a sense, a continuation of the therapy, reflecting the same values that he was seeking to bring into the therapeutic relationship. He liked to include something from the previous session, a way of maintaining empathy through the written word. He also knew that he didn't have any free appointment slots the following Monday, and then it was the May bank holiday the next week, and he didn't think it would be helpful to only offer an appointment in three weeks' time. So he decided on a time the following Wednesday when he was also at the surgery.

Dear Gary,

Sorry not to see you this morning, hope you're OK and that you're not ill. Having not heard from you I am unsure whether or not you want to continue with the counselling. I know how it can feel strange at first. I would certainly be happy to see you again and to offer you time to talk things through further.

I do accept that you don't see yourself as having a problem with drinking and I was struck by your saying how you sometimes wished you could go out for a few beers and not have any hassle, while at the same time having a sense that getting into fights was also part of how it was, how it is. I'm sure you know what you want.

Anyway, I'd be happy to see you again. I'll make a provisional appointment next week, Wednesday 30th April at 9.30 am here at the surgery.

If you have decided not to continue then please let the surgery know, but I hope to see you next Wednesday.

Regards

Rick Allen

cc Dr James

Counselling session 3: the therapeutic relationship begins to develop

Wednesday 30 April

The phone rang in the counselling room; it was Julie on reception. 'Hi Rick, Gary's here, he's not looking too good.'

'OK, thanks, I'll be along.' Not looking too good. What has happened? He hoped Gary was OK, but wondered what might have happened. Did he look unwell? He didn't know. He got up, took a quick look around the counselling room to check everything was OK, and headed down the corridor to the waiting area.

As he walked in he saw Gary sitting with his head down.

'Gary?'

Gary heard his name and looked up, and got to his feet, well, dragged himself to his feet. He felt sore, his ribs were still giving him jip. And his jaw felt tight. He only looked up briefly as he walked towards Rick.

'Good to see you, come on through.'

Gary didn't say anything, but followed Rick along the corridor to the counselling room. He sat himself down in the same chair that he had used the first time he'd come. He winced again as he sat down, trying to avoid jerking his ribs.

Rick now had more of a chance to see Gary. His face looked bruised and he had a cut on his cheek, just above his lower jaw, which had been stitched up, and his forehead was marked as well. His right eye was puffy too and a bit discoloured.

'You look as though you've had a bit of hassle.' Rick used the language that Gary had used that previous session.

'Yeah . . . yeah, you could say that.' He didn't feel inclined to say much more.

'Mhmm. So, good to see you again, sorry you didn't make it last time, but, well . . .'

'Yeah, yeah I know. I sort of didn't see much point, you know? But, well, things have sort of changed a bit, I mean, well, I had to see the doc again and, well, he told me that I really ought to come back and see you.'

'When did you see him?'

'Monday. They told me at the hospital to make an appointment.'

'You were in the hospital?'

'Up at casualty Friday night, getting stitched up.'

'So things happened Friday night.'

'Yeah.' Gary didn't nod. Head movements were still uncomfortable. 'Yeah.'

Rick was listening to Gary and observing him as well; he'd clearly been in some kind of altercation with someone, but he wasn't going to probe him on it. It wasn't the way he worked as a person-centred counsellor. It would have been to satisfy his own curiosity and that would not be responsive to what his client might want to say. Gary had made it, OK, at the urging of his doctor once again.

'Can't have been easy to get here, you look as if you'd be better off in bed, taking it easy.'

'Yeah, that's true enough. It was bad, you know, things really got out of control.'

'With what happened to you?'

'Yeah.'

Rick realised he had not empathised with the loss of control and wanted to convey that he had heard that. 'Mhmm, things got out of control.' In the light of how much Gary had emphasised not having a problem with controlling his drinking, it seemed somehow to be a comment that needed to be heard, although quite what the 'things really got out of control' applied to he knew he did not know.

'Just trying to have a few beers, you know, me and my mates. We were at a bar in town, Friday night. It was busy, always is, you know. We were there, just having a laugh, like. Anyway, this guy appears with his mates – I'd had some hassle with him a week ago. Anyway, he started having a go at me. Started to wind me up. I'd sorted him that last time, I suppose because he had his mates with him he felt brave enough to take me on.'

'Mhmm, so, someone you'd had hassle with before, only this time he was with his own mates, yeah?'

'We had words, you know. But that wasn't enough for him. I was actually feeling good, and just wanted to be left alone. But I wasn't going to put up with him mouthing off. He needed sorting out, yeah?'

'Mhmm, that's how you felt, you weren't going to put up with him, how he was behaving towards you, he needed sorting out.'

'So, yeah, well, his mates also started to have a go as well and, well, we all ended up getting thrown out of the place. They were still having a go. Fuckers. Anyway, one of them threw a bottle at Mal, caught him on the side of the head.' Gary tapped his own head to indicate where it had hit him. 'I wasn't putting up with that. I piled in, so did Luke. Mal was bleeding but, well, that didn't stop him. I fell over and got a kicking. Did my ribs, and, yeah, someone had called the police, we heard the sirens and, well, they ran off. I wasn't in a state to run anywhere. We got taken up to casualty, Mal had to have stitches, Luke was OK. He can really look after himself, we all can, I was unlucky, tripped up. Lost my balance, you know?'

'Mhmm, lost your balance.'

'Probably had had one too many, yeah.'

'Drank a bit too much to keep your balance.'

'Yeah. Yeah, well, the nurse who stitched me up had a go. Asked me what had happened, stuff like that, how often I got into trouble. I'd said that it happened, but she kept saying I was lucky, that once I was down, well, I could have got a kick in the head and there could have been real damage. She told me a bit about other guys she'd seen.'

An intervention such as this can be helpful. There is a strong case to have people trained to offer what are termed 'brief interventions' and motivational interviewing, in settings such as accident and emergency suites, and for there to be access to trained alcohol counsellors/nurses. Both brief interventions (Bien *et al*, 1993; Wilk *et al*, 1997; Poikolainen, 1999; Beich *et al*, 2003) and motivational interviewing (Miller and Rollnick, 1991) aim to promote change, to direct the client towards seeing that they have a problem and that they need to make changes in order to address it.

Such approaches contrast with the person-centred approach in which the therapist does not bring an intention to direct or encourage the client towards a specific change. The person-centred therapist recognises the working of the actualising tendency, and seeks to facilitate this internal impulse towards constructive personality change through working to create a therapeutic relationship characterised by the 'necessary and sufficient conditions' described in the Introduction. This is what makes the person-centred approach radically different. It is non-directive therapy and a fundamentally *relational therapy*. We might say that the person- or client-centred therapeutic process emerges out of the *relational experience*. Indeed, we might take this further, and go so far as to say that the person- or client-centred therapeutic process *is* the relational experience that is created between client and counsellor.

Having said that, the intention here is not to question or cast doubt on the effectiveness of brief intervention and motivational interviewing, or

> any other response to a client with an alcohol problem. It is simply to
> clarify how the person-centred approach differs fundamentally. In the
> final analysis what matters most is that clients with alcohol problems, of
> whatever age, receive the therapeutic (some would prefer to say 'treat-
> ment') responses that will most effectively offer them the opportunity
> to consider and work towards the possibility of greater wellbeing in
> their lives.

'I told her I could look after myself, you know? She said she believed me, but also
said that if I am so good at looking after myself why was I there getting stitched
up and having X-rays on my ribs.'

'Fair point. How was it hearing that?'

'Pissed me off. But . . . , yeah, well, she was sort of right in a way. I mean, yeah, I
was unlucky to trip, you know, just one of those things.'

'One of those things.'

'Drank a bit too much.'

Yeah, that's how it can be, yeah?'

'Yeah, and well, I had to see the doc yesterday, have the stitches out. He had a go
as well.'

'That how it felt, that they both had a go?'

'Well, yeah, sort of. I mean, the nurse, I mean, she was good, I liked her. I mean,
she didn't sort of have a go, but she sort of, well, made me think about what had
happened. I mean, well, yeah, she was good, I guess. I wasn't too good, still a bit
pissed though I'd begun to sober up a bit. I remember her asking me whether it
was all worth it, how many times this kind of thing was going to happen, would
I be as "lucky" next time. I told her I was just unlucky, didn't really want to
hear her. She seemed to have all this stuff in her head about alcohol. Spent a
lot of time Saturday in bed, sleeping and thinking. Wanting to get hold of
those bastards, and just wanting to not have hassle all the time as well. Seems
like every time we go out something happens.'

'Mhmm, every time you and your mates go out for a drink, it ends up going violent, you mean?'

'It does, Fridays and Saturdays – well, those are the nights we go out regularly,
can't afford it every night, you know? Wish I could, maybe one day when I can
earn a bit more.'

Rick nodded, feeling a wave of sadness that this was the goal in Gary's life,
earn more money so he could drink more, and probably end up in more
fights with more risk of damaging himself. And yet it was clearly not what
Gary was experiencing. It was one of those moments in which he knew his
own internal experience was so different from what his client was communicating. His thoughts went back to being congruent, being transparent,
being himself with his client. He allowed his internal feelings to shape
his response.

'You kind of see that as a sort of goal, earn more, drink more?'

'Well, yeah, that's what people do. People at work, they're out drinking more than I can afford. I suppose I could drink stronger drinks, get pissed quicker, I do that sometimes, but I like a few beers too even though they're not as strong.'

'So you like a few beers, OK, but they don't get you pissed like spirits will, and sometimes you just want to get pissed, yeah?'

Gary nodded. That was pretty much how it was.

Rick was conscious of not knowing how much Gary actually drank. He was conscious that they had not talked about that in the first session, but he had not directly introduced it then, the focus seemed to be elsewhere. This session felt as though it had started in a different place. He kept it in mind.

> The person-centred therapist is placing emphasis on relationship building, and is not directing the client to disclose specific information, which is in accord with the principles of person-centred working. If the client wants the therapist to know how much they are drinking, then they can disclose this, but it is not going to be sought after.

'But you're not out drinking every night?'

'Nah, though I have a few bottles at home in the week, I mean, you know, after a hard day's graft.'

'Sure, your work is quite heavy going?' Rick realised immediately that he had only responded to the work aspect of what Gary had said. His empathy was incomplete, but Gary was responding before he had a chance to add to what he had said.

'Well, no, not that bad, I work for one of the mobile phone companies, in one of the local shops. It's OK, we have a few laughs, it's a steady job, but I could do with a bit more dosh. I do a bit of overtime sometimes, should have been in on Saturday but, well, and now I'm off sick, doctor signed me off, told me to rest. Can't lift things or move around too easily with my ribs the way they are. The boss seems OK about it. So I guess I'm OK for now, but don't want to be off too long. He'll start to get the hump, know what I mean?'

'One of the risks, yeah, of getting into fights.'

'Yeah, well, suppose so. But I can handle it.'

'You can handle the effects of getting into fights, you mean?'

'Yeah, and my drinking. Though that nurse really gave me earache over it. Asked me what I drank, how much, all kinds of stuff. Didn't tell her, didn't want to get into all of that, get more grief probably.'

'So, you sort of didn't tell her how much you drank, then, didn't want to get grief over it?'

'That's right. Well, I felt sort of uncomfortable.'

'Makes you feel uncomfortable having to think about it.'

'Look, you know, I'm not an alcy.'

'Sure, I know, I hear you, Gary. You're not an alcy.' Rick paused, a slight hesitation but he could feel the words he wanted to say arising within him, and they were a true expression of what he was feeling, 'and you do drink a lot when you drink at weekends'.

'Sure, but that's normal. Everyone has a bit more at weekends, you know?'

'Everyone?'

'Yeah, the bars are packed, everyone's there, you know?'

'Mhmm, feels like everyone's there, packed in, drinking.'

'It's what you do.'

'It's what weekends are all about, yeah?'

'I work hard, I deserve it, have a few laughs, have a shag, you know, yeah, that's what it's about.'

'Mhmm, and that's what you want, a few beers, a few laughs, have a shag and feel good about it all, yeah, leaves you feeling good?'

Gary nodded, but in his head he was thinking of how he felt at the moment. Shit weekend, he thought to himself. Should have dealt with that bastard the first time, then he'd have thought twice about coming back and having a go with his mates.

'Ye-ah . . . , yeah.'

Rick heard the hesitancy in Gary's voice. 'You sound a bit unsure.'

'Well, yeah, I mean, it would be good not to have hassle, it would.'

'Just have those few beers and it not get out of control, you mean?'

'Yeah, that's right.' He looked down, feeling like he didn't want to say anything more. Truth was, he sort of didn't always like what happened, he did get fed up with it all, but what else was there to do? Friday night, Saturday night, you headed up town, that's how it was. There wasn't any thought of doing anything else, that was what you did. But a quiet drink had its appeal sometimes . . . 'Yeah, sometimes it would be good to do something different, you know?'

'Something different, no hassle, yeah?'

Gary nodded and lapsed into silence.

> The counsellor's empathic responding has enabled the client to feel heard, maybe relax a little, allowing another aspect of his experiencing to be present in his awareness – the part of him that doesn't want the hassle, but which has less voice and influence over the actual behaviour that Gary pursues. By responding to the hesitancy, the counsellor has offered that part an opportunity to become visible, to speak, to be validated.

Rick sat and waited to see if Gary wanted to say anything else. It felt as though Gary had painted a pretty clear picture of his drinking style, and clearly there was some uncertainty, hesitancy, maybe discomfort, he wasn't sure. But at the moment it seemed that it wasn't dominant enough to force a change in behaviour. And Rick wasn't going to start pushing, that wasn't his role. He was there to form a therapeutic relationship – be open and honest with Gary, try to understand him and his world, and accept him for how he was, and how he felt he needed to be. Part of Gary wanted less hassle, and having voiced it, he felt that this was probably what was now in Gary's thoughts. He respected his client's silence. It enabled Gary to remain connected with whatever had become present in his awareness.

Gary was sitting and continuing to stare down at the carpet. Yeah, he thought, less hassle, a break from it all. He'd just moved and his ribs were sore. He tried to free himself up a bit, he was stiff, and got a shooting pain for his troubles. 'Fuck,' he muttered under his breath.

'In pain?'

'Yeah, bastards.' As far as Gary was concerned it was their fault, not his, they'd given him the kicking. His only fault was that he'd stumbled.

'Bastards?'

'The ones who did it.'

Rick nodded. 'Mhmm, bastards for giving you a good kicking, yeah?'

'Won't happen again.'

'Mhmm, you're clear on that, yeah?'

Gary nodded.

'I guess I'm wondering how you'll make sure it doesn't happen again.'

'I won't fall over.'

'Simple as that, huh, won't fall over?'

Gary looked up. 'You don't think I can stay on my own feet?'

'Reality is you weren't able to.'

Rick returned Gary's eye contact. It felt a bit like that first session when there had been some eye contact. For Gary there was an awareness again that Rick seemed solid, didn't seem phased by anything. But it pissed him off as well.

'Just will.'

'Mhmm, I hope so. It's a bugger going out drinking and getting into fights when part of yourself just wants a few quiet beers without hassle.'

This response might be characterised as 'delayed empathy' or a kind of 'reflective empathy', focused not so much on what has been said, but on the relationship between what has been said, the contrast of wanting one thing but getting something else. Rick is letting Gary know that he has heard this contrast and that, as he says, 'it's a bugger'. Rick's intention is to convey empathy. Had he been saying this in order to make Gary see it like this, or see it in a particular way, then the response would have not been in accord with person-centred therapy, it would have been an attempt to direct the client to see something from the perspective of the counsellor's frame of reference.

'Yeah, too right. It's not that I go looking for trouble, you know, it just happens.'

'Mhmm, just happens, you don't sort of look for it.'

'Well, you know,' Gary tried to grin, it was painful, it ended up as a grimace, 'maybe I do, I mean, people irritate me, you know. They knock into you, look at you, they piss me off.'

'Feels like, what, they sort of get to you.'

They're in my space, in my face, yeah ... Ahh, I don't know.' He thought for a moment

'You don't know?'

'Ah they just . . . , it's hard to explain, I just get wound up, and it's sort of, yeah, it's sort of a good feeling, place is heaving, music's loud, you're feeling good, and, well, yeah, you're up for it.'

'OK, let me check I'm getting this, you're in a packed bar, say, loud music, you've had a few drinks, and you're feeling good, and at the same time you're feeling, what you call "up for it", yeah?'

'Well, yeah, you're sort of looking out, you know. It's like you start having a look around the place, get a feel for what's going on, then, well, you kind of have your drinks and then, yeah, you sort of, I don't know, feel different.'

'So, after a few beers in that environment, you begin to feel kind of different in some way?'

Gary nodded. 'Yeah, it's like, I don't know, different, yeah.'

'Different, and it's kind of hard to sort of describe what that "different" is like, yeah?'

Gary had lifted his arms by his sides, his fists clenched slightly.

Rick reflected his arm and hand movements. It felt to him like the kind of movement you might make before punching someone. He wondered how much the body movements were capturing the flavour of what the 'difference' was.

Empathy is not only about words. Body movement can also convey that the counsellor has heard/received something that is being communicated by the client through their body. Seeing someone adopt a posture that you, as a client, are adopting as an expression of something you feel, in a sense is an opportunity to look in a mirror, to see yourself and to experience yourself in the same moment. The counsellor may not need to say anything, the movement or posture will be speaking its own language.

Gary noted Rick's response, and he nodded slightly, seeing the tightness in Rick's body. 'yeah, it's like you sort of feel wound up, tight, you know?'

'Tight, what, in your body, you mean?'

'Yeah and, well, I mean, it's like things sort of, I don't know, it feels like . . . ,' Gary couldn't find the words to describe it. 'There's a lot going on.'

'Mhmm, that's how it feels when it happens, yeah, there's a lot going on.'

'It's like, yeah, and I get irritated, pissed off with people.'

'OK, that's clear, when it's like that you're feeling irritated and pissed off with people, you mean the people around you?'

'Yeah. It's like you're sort of more aware of everyone. I mean, it's OK if it's a girl that's close, but it's usually guys, you know? At least, that's how it feels. Just gets to me.'

'Something about it all gets to you. And you've had a few drinks, and the place
    has presumably got more packed since you went in?'
'Oh yeah, I mean, we get there I guess a bit ahead of the rush, easier to get to the
    bar, you know? But yeah, it's when it gets busy and, yeah, my head's starting to
    buzz a bit.'
'OK, your head is buzzing, people are jammed in, it's noisy and there something
    about what's happening that leaves you pissed off and irritated.'
'And, yeah, yeah, and that's when, well, you know, when something sort of
    happens.'
'Mhmm, OK, that's when you feel yourself sort of, what did you say earlier, "up
    for it", yeah?'
'Yeah, yeah that's right.'
'And you want to go out to the bar, but you say you just want a few quiet beers?'
'Yeah, sometimes, but, well, yeah, it's also good to be in there with everyone, just
    pisses me off as well, winds me up.'
'This may sound a weird question but I'm trying to get a feel for what it's like, but
    do you kind of enjoy feeling wound up?'
'It's sort of part of it, you know?'
'Part of being out, part of the experience, you mean?'
'Yeah, I guess so, but it sort of, I don't know, Mal and Luke'll say to me that, well,
    they can sort of sense a change in me.'

An important disclosure. Gary acknowledges that he changes and that it is
perceived by others too. The client is showing signs of being open to explore
an experience that he would previously not have been ready to make the
counsellor aware of, or indeed to fully engage with himself. The openness
in the therapeutic relationship, the fact that Gary feels heard, respected,
taken seriously, is enabling him to disclose more, bring more of himself and
how he experiences himself into the therapeutic relationship.

'What, they tell you at the time?'
'No, no, usually later, I mean, you know, sometimes we'll talk about what's hap-
    pened, another evening maybe. Not at the time, you can't really talk much,
    music's too loud, and everyone's talking and you know, that's how it is.'
For Rick it felt awful. It certainly wasn't an experience that he personally felt any
    urge to engage with.
'So, at some time later they may tell you that they sensed something change
    in you.'
'They say I sort of look around more, sort of stare in a different kind of way.'
'Mhmm, OK, so they can see a change, and you sort of feel it in terms of irritation
    and being pissed off with people – and they see it in terms of how you look?'
Gary nodded. 'Yeah. So what's that about?'
Rick nodded slowly. 'It gets to you, doesn't it? Whether it's primarily the noise,
    the people, the alcohol, or something else, it gets to you and you sort of go

into some other sort of state in yourself, and that's when things can happen, when something might happen that'll trigger off or lead to a fight or an argument or something like that.'

Rather than a simple empathic response acknowledging the question, the therapist has got himself into a monologue. Although it has value as a kind of summary, it is reinforcing the therapist as 'the expert', the one who knows and understands and can explain what is happening for Gary. It is not a person-centred response.

The client then takes this as meaning that he is not what he terms 'an alcy', which is an agenda that the client has in order to maintain his self-concept.

'So I'm not an alcy?'
'No, you're not an alcy, you simply find yourself reacting in a particular way to a particular set of experiences and part of that is that you've been drinking.'

Rick might have responded with, 'that's really important, not being an alcy', assuming he sensed the importance and it wasn't a meaning that he was introducing from his own frame of reference.

Gary thought about what Rick had said. It did seem to sum it up. He'd never really talked to anyone quite like this before, not about himself and certainly not about this kind of thing. It wasn't something you did. Yet somehow it felt sort of . . . , yeah, it left him kind of curious to sort of know more.
'If I wasn't there, then I wouldn't react like that, do you mean?'
'I don't know. Is that how it is? Do you only get like that in that kind of experience?'
'Pretty much. I mean, you know, I can feel pissed off at home, at work, yeah, but nothing like I do when I'm out like that.'
'And what about when you drink at other times?'
'Yeah, I can sort of lose it a bit if I drink too much at a party, say, or at home sometimes, yeah, it can happen, but not always, you know?'
Rick nodded. He felt good that he and Gary seemed to be communicating and it felt quite open. He didn't feel that Gary was being defensive in any way, he seemed more able to say things as they were. That was encouraging. He'd accepted that he could lose it when drinking.
'OK, so when you drink at a party or at home, sometimes, not all of the time but sometimes you can lose it and does that mean it's sort of similar to how it is in the bar?'
'How d'you mean?'
'How it feels.'
Gary thought about it. It wasn't easy. 'Similar but different.'

'So it's sort of similar but it feels different as well in some way.'

'I'm not so irritated, not so wound up. But I do get sort of, well, people say I get angry, and, yeah, I do.'

'Angry, and do you feel that in the bar or at a club?'

'Yeah, yeah I get angry when people piss me off.'

'So in the bar it's people pissing you off that makes you angry, at home or at a party it might be something else?'

'I don't know. I just get angry sometimes, you know?'

'It's sort of there.'

'Yeah, makes me want to sort of lash out, or give someone some verbal.'

'Yeah, you get angry and you want to say or do something with it, lash out, give someone some verbal, that kind of thing, yeah?'

'Yeah, that's right.' Gary lapsed into silence. His mind had drifted back into the past, to scenes and sounds from his early childhood. He pushed them aside. Yeah, so he got angry. He'd got reason to be angry. And besides, there were people out there that pissed him off.

Memories emerge within the session. These are not new memories that are breaking into awareness for the first time. They are familiar to the client, though they are emerging into awareness within the counselling session for the first time. The client, however, does not want them, and pushes them away. Nevertheless, the fact of connecting with something deep makes an impact on the therapeutic relationship. Rick feels a change and he chooses to voice what he is experiencing.

Rick felt a shift in atmosphere, it seemed as though Gary had sort of suddenly become a little bit distant. It was as though his client had gone somewhere within himself and he felt that he had been sort of left behind. He trusted these experiences, they often indicated that a client had momentarily engaged with a part of themselves or of their experience that was in some way hidden, or had not been revealed, or something deep with significant feelings associated with it. He wondered what Gary might have been experiencing. He acknowledged the moment to himself and noted that Gary seemed to look distant as well. It felt very present.

'You look suddenly distant.'

'Hmm, oh, yeah, thinking about stuff.' Gary noticed that his heart had started thumping, he wasn't sure what that was about. He wasn't going to say anything about what he'd been thinking. He didn't want to. That was past, he'd dealt with that, it just came back at him sometimes.

'Mhmm, stuff.'

'Yeah, you know, the past.' He glanced at the clock, not much time left. 'Anyway, nearly time to go.'

'Yeah. Anything else you want to say before you head off, and do you want to come again in a week or two?'

> No pressure is put on the client to disclose the 'stuff'. Gary is allowed to keep his power, maintain a course of action that he wants to take. Rick is communicating that he has heard that there is stuff but that he is not going to force disclosure. It creates the possibility for Gary to realise that he can say things and there won't be pressure to take it further if he doesn't want to. He has control, it is not threatened or being taken away from him.

'Yeah, yeah it's sort of made more sense this week. It's felt OK,' though as he spoke he could feel his heart thumping. He didn't know why, didn't see any connection. The past was the past. He had to get on with the present.

'Mhmm, feeling OK, made more sense.'

'Yeah.' He paused. 'But I've got to get myself sorted, you know. It's OK off work but it's boring, you know? Particularly when you can't move around too easily. I don't want to be off work like this too long, drives me crazy.'

'So, boring and drive you crazy, huh, being off work like this?'

'Hopefully not for too long. Stitches out tomorrow, they want to see me back at the hospital for that. I'm signed off for two weeks, doctor wants me to have time for my rib to heal. I'm all strapped up under here to stop me moving too much. Can I come back next week, while I'm off, it's sort of easier.'

'Sure. Can't be Monday, bank holiday, but next Wednesday, same time, that's fine.'

'OK. And sorry about last time, I just, well, just didn't see any point in coming. I sort of feel different somehow today.' He'd pushed his memories aside and his heart wasn't thumping now in quite the same way. He felt more focused, more himself.

'Sure, but if you don't think you're going to make it, you could let us know at the surgery, yeah?'

Gary nodded, 'Yeah, OK.'

The session ended and Gary left. His heart had settled down again and he really didn't think any more of it. He knew what he'd had to cope with in the past, but he had done just that, coped. It wasn't a problem. And, yeah, people did get to him, he could get angry, but lots of people were like that. It wasn't a problem. It wasn't a problem.

Rick was sitting reflecting on the session. He felt a kind of connection with Gary. He could really begin to get a feel for Gary's life – not all of it, he'd only been shown some parts of it. But that last session there had been times when he had felt more connected, what was it Rogers had written, about being integrated into the relationship? Yes, that felt more the case than the first session.

> The third necessary and sufficient condition for constructive personality change as defined by Rogers runs, 'the second person, whom we shall term the therapist, is congruent or integrated in the relationship' (Rogers, 1957a, p.96). To be congruent or integrated into the relationship is

concerned with presence, with how present the therapist is, with how much of the therapist as a person is accurately present and available to, and within, the therapeutic relationship.

He wondered about what happened for Gary after a few beers. Was it just the surroundings, or was it primarily the alcohol getting to him? He realised that he again had said nothing about safe drinking. But he was OK with that. For now his role was to establish the therapeutic relationship. If and when they got into the specifics of how much Gary was drinking then it would be more timely. He guessed that maybe the nurse at the accident and emergency department may have said something, and most probably his GP. He knew that it was a very relevant topic in that environment and that there were various initiatives around the country to target young binge drinkers when they attended an accident and emergency department for their injuries.

Government guidelines in the UK suggest that safe drinking is up to 3–4 units of alcohol a day for men and 2–3 units of alcohol a day for women, and no bingeing (six units or more at a time).

Points for discussion

- How has your sense of Gary's inner world developed from reading this session?
- Evaluate Rick's responses. How has he communicated his warm acceptance of Gary?
- Were there times when you felt you would have responded differently and, if so, what response would you have made and why?
- How did you feel about Rick's letter to Gary? Would you have said more or less, or approached the situation in a different way?
- What would you take to supervision from this session?

Write notes for this session.

CHAPTER 3

Supervision session 1: impressions explored and a matter of congruence

Friday 9 May

Rick had been discussing two of his other clients with Jean, his supervisor. He now turned his attention to Gary.

'Now, I've got another new client at the surgery. Young man, 18, referred by the doctor, getting into fights linked to his drinking. He hasn't said anything about his home life, and really he's focused mainly on his experiences of drinking and, well, persuading me that he hasn't got a problem, that he's "not an alcy". That seems really important for him to keep saying, and I don't know why, I don't know if that has any specific meaning for him, or if it is more of a general comment.'

'So, he doesn't want to think of himself as an "alcy", I wonder what he means by that?'

'He referred to the people who drink down by the river in town.'

'OK.'

'And he talks about being able to control his drinking as well, that seems important. And then, well, after the first session, he then didn't show for the second two weeks later, and then came in on Wednesday. He'd been in a fight, got himself beaten up a bit – cracked ribs – he never said how many – cut on his face that had to be stitched and a bit bruised and battered. But it was actually a session where I felt more connected – except for one time when he seemed to drift off into his own thoughts momentarily, and then came back, and I haven't a clue what that was about. But there's something, something not right, something missing. I don't know what it is.' Rick paused before continuing. 'He gets angry, he gets irritated and pissed off with people, usually in bars when it's crowded and he's been drinking.'

'Angry young man, then, not sure why, but alcohol's in the frame.'

Rick nodded.

'And you, how does it feel being there with him?'

'Felt a bit uneasy I guess at first. No, that's not the right word, took a while to sort of get going. He was there because the doctor had told him to come, but Gary didn't – and doesn't – think he has an alcohol problem. So it felt a bit cat and mouse, I suppose, because he clearly does, it's causing him problems, but whether it's the primary cause or there is something else driving his need to drink, to fight, that's the unknown.'

'But you're already thinking that way?'

'I know some people just get into fights simply because alcohol seems to affect them that way, but often there are underlying factors, frustrations, maybe exposure to violence themselves, and besides, kids, young people, are exposed to so much more violence these days on TV, or so it seems to me. I don't know, but I sense something. And, yeah, in that first session there is something about him. He's not exactly big, but not small, average I guess, but there's a sort of attitude and, well, a feeling that he can flip into a side of himself that is maybe different. I don't know, it's all a bit hazy, but I just have a sense of something. At the moment it feels really important to build the therapeutic relationship, really let him know that I am there to understand, to accept him as he is, as he needs to be, and to be straight with him as well. It's so important and I wonder how many people don't have this experience in their lives, and how it affects them. And how has Gary been affected by, perhaps shaped by is a better way of expressing it, how has Gary been shaped by his life experiences to make him the person he is, and experiences himself as, today? I can see some of the effects, but I don't have the causes, and I may do, I may not. My role is to concentrate on the therapeutic relationship, and what emerges will be what needs to emerge, in its own time and in its own way.'

> The person-centred counsellor will wish to focus on being fully present and available to their client. They will wish to ensure that they maintain congruence, that their positive regard for the client is unconditional, and they will want to ensure not only that their empathy is accurate, but that it is also inclusive and not selective. Supervision is a relational experience in which the person-centred counsellor can address where they feel they may not be offering these aspects of therapeutic relationship. It is a place in which they can identify blocks to empathy and unconditional positive regard, acknowledge and explore disconnection from the client or unease or anxiety that may be emerging within them as signs of their own incongruence.

'Sure.' Jean was still with something that Rick had said previously, 'so, something about unease, and something about feeling he could flip into some other sort of part of himself in some way?'

Rick responded. 'Yes, it's like I see what I am shown, and in that first session there was a moment of sensing something, I don't know, almost sort of menacing but that feels too strong. A sort of restlessness, and readiness to lash out. He talked about that in the last session, and couldn't find the words to describe how he could feel sometimes when he gets wound up, irritated, pissed off by people. Yes, I remember he raised his arms, like this.' Rick raised his arms, fists slightly clenched. 'He couldn't find the words to convey the feelings. It was very much in his body.'

'My reaction to that is to wonder whether his language is somehow stored more in his body than in his mind, if that makes any sense.'

'That's interesting. I don't know. But it seemed like his body carried the sense of being wound up, but he's also talking of feeling irritated, pissed off, seems like he has a short fuse, at least he does in some situations and, it seems, that alcohol is linked to this.'

'Shortening the fuse, perhaps?'

'Could be, I don't know, but could be something like that, but, yes, interesting metaphor, but the thought has come to my mind that if alcohol shortens the fuse maybe something else lights it.'

'And when both happen . . .'

'. . . bang. Someone is going to get whacked.'

'Mhmm.'

'This is helpful. I sort of feel it's helping me to get in touch with me and with what's happening. And that metaphor really does help me although, well, obviously it's emerged here and is not something that may necessarily have meaning for Gary.'

'No, I agree, and that's important to remember, of course.'

'OK, so, if alcohol shortens the fuse then maybe it's the environment, people, what's going on around him, he seems to become sensitive to people looking at him, or being in his space, in his face, I think that was what he said. Something like that, I think.'

'So, people in his space.'

'Usually in bars, clubs, where there's a lot of energy, noise, you know?'

'Mhmm, it sort of gets to him in some way.'

'But not only there, sometimes he can get angry he said at home after a few beers, or at a party, say, though that's going to be a bit like being in a bar, of course.'

'Think he's using anything else?'

'So many young people do. I hadn't thought of that. I don't know. Maybe. Hmm. That is a thought. He hasn't said anything. Maybe he'll feel able to disclose that as the relationship develops, if that's what's happening.'

'Something to bear in mind although, yes, our role isn't to introduce our own speculations, of course. At least he is attending. You say he missed one appointment?'

'And then he came for the session after that, and wants to come next week, so I think he's feeling drawn to it. We'll have to see.'

'And given his record of fights, do you feel safe with him?'

'I don't feel he's likely to react that way to me. I've got the alarm button in the room, but I don't feel that. Yes, I can see the anger, and he doesn't like the idea of having an alcohol problem – something about that, don't know what it is. I mean, most people aren't comfortable with that, but there's an edge to it with him, it's like it's sort of even more important.'

'Particularly important to him.'

'Very much so.' Rick took a deep breath. 'Like it's sort of personal. I don't know, I'm sure I will be talking more about him next time. I'm looking forward to working with him, I feel a bit like Sherlock Holmes, in a way, not that I feel an urge to probe around, that's not what I mean, but more of a sense of being faced with a puzzle, a person for whom things aren't working out, aren't, perhaps, quite what they seem. And I don't want to go over the top on this speculation, but I am aware of having this sense of there being something else. He doesn't come across as simply the young binge drinker who is only drinking for a good time, even though that's what he says. And it's not that I don't accept what he says, I do, it's his reality, and yet . . .'

'As you say, and yet . . . It's important not to put two and two together and come up with five.'

> The person-centred approach does not require or indeed encourage the therapist to try to make sense of the client during the session. The therapist's role is straightforward (though not simple) and demanding – to offer the therapeutic conditions.

'That's right. Talking like this has helped. I really want to try and help him to work out what's happening and to, well, make choices that are perhaps less damaging – if that's what he wants. I think he does, but it's all too soon, all too uncertain, all too new to even accept to some degree that there's something problematic happening for him.'

'Yes, so a sense that time will tell, and you need to keep your focus on offering the therapeutic conditions.'

'That's right. I hope so. And I am conscious of not having made any mention of safe drinking and alcohol units, and, well, it's not exactly my role, I'm a general counsellor, but I am aware of these factors and, well, I don't think Gary has a sense that the amount he is probably drinking will take him above safe drinking simply in terms of units, let alone the impact it seems to be having on his behaviour and his perception.'

'Where does that leave you, knowing you are not introducing this information?'

'Uneasy. That word again. I don't believe in withholding something that I know the client may not be aware of. I think there is something about the quality and genuineness of my unconditional positive regard if I hold back information that is relevant to what a client is experiencing. Not that I want to in any way appear an expert, but the reality is that Gary is drinking in a way that is problematic, even though he is not making the connection . . . Hmm. And that's it, isn't it. He needs to make that connection. It probably won't be as therapeutic if I make it for him.' He paused and took another deep breath. 'And that's the tough bit.'

'Tough bit?'

'Not saying anything, while he continues to do himself damage.'

'You sound as though you are making the assumption that saying something
would make him change.'

Rick smiled. 'True, and it probably wouldn't. There are always leaflets, of course,
though maybe the doctor has already given him one? I could check that out.
But then, what would I do with what I learn from that? I've got to manage my
discomfort and, yes, I think I did say that I agreed he wasn't an alcy, but I think
I may have said that it did seem to me alcohol was causing problems. At least, I
think that's what I said, to be honest I can't remember. But that is what I'd
hope to say, be honest. Not try to change his view, but rather offer him mine
because that's what I'm sitting there thinking and feeling.'

'And that brings up the whole issue of being congruent.'

'Or transparent. And is it for me to judge what to say and when, or do I rather rely
on the experience in the moment? If I am feeling connected to my client – integrated in the relationship – and if the urge to mention something seems strong
and persistent, then I should act on it, and then check it out here, in supervision.
What I don't want is for my transparency to in some way disrupt my conveying,
and my client's perception of, empathic understanding and unconditional positive regard in the sense that I become pre-occupied with what is present for me,
rather than what is being communicated to me by him.'

The factor of intention is important. If a therapist is considering disclosing
something of their own perception towards what a client is doing, thinking
or feeling, they must consider their intention and motivation. 'Why do I
need to tell my client this, and for whose benefit is it?' It may be a genuine
offer of a piece of knowledge that the therapist is aware of and that the client
might find valuable. But it is not advice, it is not an attempt to tell the
client what to think, feel or do.

This is a difficult area, particularly where the therapist may have specialist knowledge on a topic that is relevant to what the client is exploring. However, the primary role of the therapist is to attend to the inner
world of the client. And where there is the thought to share a piece of
information, intention and motivation should be considered, at the time
and in supervision.

'Your, our, primary duty, it could be said, is to attend to the client. But you seek to
achieve this from a state of congruence, yes?'

'Yes, if I am not congruent then I would argue that my empathy and unconditional positive regard cannot be considered trustworthy. And then I am false,
unreal, and certainly not offering the possibility of a therapeutic alliance or
relationship with my client.'

'Mhmm.' Jean nodded. This was so true, and yet how many times had she heard
people say that they 'do congruence', or 'do empathy and unconditional positive regard' with no reference to how they are in that moment, the state of their
own awareness of their own experiencing? Fortunately not many who had

been trained in the approach to some depth. She brought her thoughts back to what Rick was saying. 'Hence the complex and disciplined nature of person-centred counselling and psychotherapy.'

'And I want to add "person-centred psychology" because it is a psychological system as well as a therapeutic approach.'

The person-centred approach or client-centred therapy is not often described in terms of person- or client-centred psychology. For most people person- or client-centred is associated with counselling and psychotherapy. However, it is part of the tradition of humanistic psychology. Rogers was himself a psychologist and person/client-centred theory and practice is a robust psychological system for understanding and working with psychological problems.

The session moved on to a consideration of work with another client. After the session ended Rick felt that he had somehow re-ordered his thinking, feeling and perception of Gary in some way. It felt as though he had been able to pull together some hazy and disparate strands, he felt more focused, clearer. It felt good. He was looking forward to their next session.

Counselling session 4: memories intrude, the drinking's 'not a problem'

Wednesday 7 May

'So, how're you doing?'

'Yeah, not so bad. Still stiff, but, yeah, taking it easy, you know?'

'Sure. Still having to take it easy.'

'Yeah.' Gary shook his head. 'Had a good weekend, though. Took it carefully, like, having to. Don't want to do myself more damage. Still strapped up but on the mend I guess. Going back to work next week, I reckon. Just gotta take it easy.'

'Mhmm. Taking it easy seems to be the way it has to be for you at the moment.'

Gary nodded. Yes, he thought to himself, he didn't much like it, having to rest up and stuff, he wasn't too good sitting about. Got twitchy. Liked to be on the go. Been like that for a while, well, it was how he was. He'd been watching videos at home, action movies, dramatic, violent, anything like that. Made him feel good. He liked all that. 'Yeah, gets to you, you know? Winds me up. Still, a few beers settles me down. Just having to take it easy. Can't get into fights when I'm like this.' He grinned.

'No, not in a good condition for getting into fights. So it's hard to take it easy, it winds you up and you need a drink to, what, unwind?'

'Yeah, relaxes me, you know?'

Alcohol is a relaxant. It suppresses the functioning of the nervous system, relieving natural anxieties, or reducing the tension that arises in the person who has developed some degree of dependence on anxiety – needing to maintain a certain level of alcohol in the body in order to stave off withdrawal reactions.

'Mhmm.' Rick didn't say anything further; a brief silence arose between them. It felt tense.

'It's not a problem.'

'No, no, not a problem, having a drink to settle yourself down.'

'Nurse at the hospital had another go, though. Kept telling me about how alcohol affected you. But it doesn't affect me, I'm OK.'

'Mhmm, so what she told you doesn't feel like it's affecting you at the moment, or not like she was telling you.' Rick added the 'at the moment'. That was the focus, that was where Gary's focus was centred.

'No . . . , well, no.' Gary hadn't liked what he'd been told. It wasn't something he wanted to think about too much. He'd seen his father drinking heavily, before he left. Didn't see him much now, he hated how his father had become, and he didn't want to be like that. He had no respect for him, had no respect for anyone that was an alcy. He wasn't going to be like that. He was just drinking like his mates did, that was all. Just that, well, people upset him, got on his nerves, got in his face, and it needed sorting.

Rick heard the hesitation in Gary's voice.

'You sound a bit uncertain?'

'No . . . , I mean, well, you know, kept telling me about how many people start off drinking without thinking it's going to be a problem – in fact, well, she sort of said that's how it was for everyone pretty much. How it sort of creeps up on you, suddenly you find yourself not just drinking now and then, but drinking every day, giving yourself a reason to. I mean, yeah, OK, I drink most days, but I control it. I can choose not to.'

'Mhmm, so what she said sort of got to you a bit, but you feel like you're in control, it's not going to creep up on you. That how it is?'

'Yeah.'

'And you can choose not to drink if you want to, yeah?'

'Well, yeah . . . , yeah, course I can.'

'Mhmm.' Rick paused. 'I'm unclear, are you saying that you do choose not to sometimes, or that you could choose not to if you had to or wanted to?'

'What do you mean?'

Rick realised that he'd clearly taken it too far. Now he was going to have to explain what he had said. He'd moved away from Gary's frame of reference, but he genuinely wasn't clear, and he also knew how what he'd asked could have felt more than a bit probing to Gary.

The counsellor is pushing, and there is the feel of an agenda here. So often, people do think they have control, when they don't. The counsellor is not accepting that Gary feels or at least wants to communicate that he feels able to be in control of his drinking. Gary has been quite clear, he has said that he could choose not to drink if he wanted to. The counsellor needs to ask himself why he isn't hearing what Gary is saying. The likelihood is because it is not matching his agenda. The counsellor has stepped away from the client's frame of reference, he is not accepting what the client is saying. His urge to encourage the client to recognise he has a problem is getting in the way. The person-centred approach requires the counsellor to accept what is present for the client; even if they disagree with the way the client may be interpreting an experience, their first duty is to accept the client's experiencing.

'Look, I want to be honest with you here, Gary, it feels to me like your drinking has caused you a problem, that's why you're strapped up. And I'm concerned it's going to get out of control.' Rick meant what he said, and he could feel his own emotion present as he spoke. He wasn't sure quite how Gary would experience what he had just said, or interpret it, but that was what he was feeling. It wasn't for him to try and make some excuse for what he had just been saying in response to Gary; that would just add to the incongruence that had emerged in their relationship. Better to be clear and open, transparent, and then the client can have a free and open choice as to how he then wants to respond to what has been communicated.

Gary listened. Rick sounded pretty clear, he didn't sound like a counsellor, more like, well, like a mate, sort of. He wasn't, but he sounded different.

'You mean that?'

Rick nodded. 'I do. And I do hear what you're saying as well.'

But you don't agree?'

'It's not how I see it, but it is how you do. I let my concern get in the way of hearing what you were saying about feeling able to choose.'

Gary took a deep breath. 'Well, yeah. I mean. You know, it's not a problem. Shit, why does everyone think I have a problem?'

'That must be how it feels, everyone thinks you've got a problem.'

Gary's thoughts went briefly back to his father. How he hated him, how he was when he'd been drinking, crashing about, swearing, shouting, it had been really scary at times. And there'd been the violence as well ... He was quite caught up in his memories, almost oblivious for a few moments to being in the counselling room. He would never be like him. Never ... never.

Rick felt the quiet in the room, there had been sudden change of atmosphere. He knew from experience how this could be indicative of something significant happening. Gary was sitting silently staring down, his face in a fixed expression, almost devoid of emotion. He did not know what he was experiencing and he wasn't going to sit there speculating to himself. He needed to keep his focus, even though nothing was being said. He needed to keep his attention on Gary and maintain his sense of warmth towards him. What had been the last thing he had said? About how it must feel that everyone thinks he's got a problem. It had seemed as though Gary was going to release a burst of anger and then . . . , then this silence.

Gary continued to sit, the intensity of the memory had passed. Now he just sat, not sure what to say. He knew he was OK, he wasn't like *him*. He would never be like that. He just liked to be sociable, have a few laughs, yeah, and if things got a bit 'difficult', he sorted it out. Nothing wrong with that. That wasn't a problem; he looked after himself, that was what it was all about, you looked after yourself and your mates and, yeah, they looked out for you. That was how it was. Wasn't a problem. None of it was a problem. Just a laugh, yeah, that's what it was. Just a laugh . . .

The client is denying the reality of his drinking and its effects to himself, because of what it might mean. He cannot risk allowing himself to see his drinking as in any way being a problem. He has created a self-concept of not being like his father, a kind of internal imperative. He has to maintain this self-concept; his identity is at stake, or so it feels. He may not be consciously thinking of it like this, but a kind of internal incongruence is present. His way of dealing with it is to deny to his experience the possibility of his having a problem with alcohol. Thereby he can preserve his self-concept. To do otherwise would be too painful, too psychologically devastating at this time to countenance.

The person-centred counsellor would want the client to acknowledge that he has a problem when he is able, when his own internal process allows this. The client's process of being is trusted. The person-centred therapist does not intentionally force incongruent experiencing or functioning to the surface, into awareness, but it can and does happen as a result of the therapeutic experience. The seven stages in the process of change that takes a person from incongruence to greater congruence and to fuller functionality as a person are described by Rogers (1967a, pp.125–59), and have been outlined in the Introduction of this volume.

Rick noticed the expression on Gary's face change, he could see a slight smile.

'Yeah, not a problem. I take care of things . . .' He paused and stretched, realising he hadn't moved for a while, and as he did so he felt pain in his ribs. 'Fuck!'

Rick saw the grimace on Gary's face. 'Painful, huh?'

'Too fucking right. Shit.' He moved his back, trying to straighten it a little. He felt stiff. 'It gets like this. You just have to put up with it. Doc says it'll sort itself out, just have to take it easy.'

'Mhmm, take it easy.' Rick nodded and imagined that probably he looked sympathetic. Gary did look in pain.

For some reason Gary's thoughts were back with his father. He didn't really
want to think about him. He'd pissed off, good riddance. It had been tough,
yeah, course it had, but they'd managed. Yeah, he didn't want to think
about him. Just wanted to get on with his life. He sighed, he wasn't sure
why, he just did.

Rick noticed and responded to it. 'Makes you sigh, yeah?'

Gary nodded. 'Yeah.' He snorted. 'Yeah, fucking mystery.'

'Mhmm, something a fucking mystery.'

Gary shook his head. 'My old man, fuck's sake, he was a drunken bastard, fucking
alcy. Fucked me up, you know, and mum.'

'Feels like he fucked you and your mum up.'

'Getting pissed, crashing about, beat mum up a few times, had a go at me as well.
I'd hide when he came in.'

Rick was aware of not knowing how old Gary had been when this had been happening, but he didn't need to know. He'd find out if and when Gary wanted to
tell him. He responded with empathy. 'So, he'd be violent to you and your
mum. Made you want to hide from him.'

Gary nodded. 'Yeah. That's how he'd be. And then, another time, he'd be all, I
don't know, sort of tell you everything was OK. He'd sort of get all tearful.'
Gary shook his head. 'I hated that. Well, I hated it all, but he'd sort of, you
know, I mean I'd hear him, telling my mum he was sorry, it'd be different
now, all that crap. And she'd believe him.' He shook his head. 'Don't understand that. But I guess she couldn't throw him out. And I wasn't old enough.
I probably would now, I'd have a go at him, that's for sure. But . . . , well, you
know, what was I, nine, ten. Just kept out of the way.'

'Mhmm, so you'd throw him out now, but then you were nine or ten and kept
away from him.'

'Tried to. Tried to.' Gary lapsed back into silence and Rick felt the atmosphere
change again in the room, in the relationship.

He responded quietly not wanting to disturb whatever was happening for Gary.
'Tried to keep away from him.' He waited to see how Gary would respond.

This is a very human moment. The client is connecting at depth to feelings
and memories that, as they emerge into awareness, take on a reality in the
present. Material is being disclosed that lies at the core of much of the difficulties Gary is facing in the present. He discloses that his father clearly had
an alcohol problem, contributing to his violent behaviour towards Gary and
his mother. This is a significant time in the therapeutic process as more of
Gary's previously hidden experiences are made visible to Rick, offering the
opportunity for Gary to receive empathic understanding and unconditional
positive regard. In other words, Gary's painful memories, the feelings and
thoughts that are associated with what happened to him, emerge and are
communicated to Rick. As a result, and while experiencing what has

become present for him, Gary is offered the experience of a warm, accepting and compassionate response from another human being. In a sense, in a very real sense, this human-to-human, person-to-person moment heralds the start of a healing process.

Gary's jaw was firm as he thought back to the past, and felt his body tense. His old man'd been out of order. Sometimes, just sometimes, it did trouble him, just slightly, when he thought about the fights he'd been in, but then, well, he knew they were different, people out of order, in his face, in his space. They were different. Yeah, he lost it sometimes, course he did, people do, that's how it is. But he never really lost control, not really. He did what he had to do. People would irritate him when he was out drinking. He didn't like it and he wasn't one to hesitate in sorting out something, or someone, he didn't like. What was it Rick had just said? Oh yeah, keeping away from his old man. Yeah. Yeah, but if he tried anything now, he'd go for him, he knew that. He could feel it inside him, the tension in his body.

The client feels violent towards his father, but in having these feelings he must not allow them to cause him to in any way identify with his father's behaviour. He has to see his own violence or urge to violence as being different, in order to preserve his self-concept.

Rick could see how tense Gary was as he sat there. His arms were tight, his fists clenched. He looked like he was ready to explode, or that he could do. He guessed it was linked to his father. He didn't say anything, letting Gary be as he was.

Yeah, thought Gary, I'd punch his lights out now, and he knew that he could. There wasn't any respect for his father. He'd lost that a long time ago. He didn't want to know him, and was glad he didn't have contact with him. He could imagine himself punching him down and giving him a good kicking, let him know what it could feel like. Fuck him, he thought to himself.

Rick continued to sit, aware that the silence was feeling more intense, and very aware that Gary seemed set in the chair, not moving, locked into whatever thought process was present for him. His body still looked tense, his fists still clenched, the muscles in his arms tight. 'Your body looks tense, tight.'

Gary heard Rick's voice. Yes, yes it was, he thought to himself. It often was. A few drinks relaxed him though. He could count on that. 'Yeah, well, gets to you, you know?'

'The memories, you mean?'

Gary nodded and relaxed slightly. 'Yeah, does my head in sometimes, need to relax, you know, few beers, that helps.'

'Mhmm, few beers helps you to relax, yeah, unwind?'

Gary nodded, aware as well that, yeah, it did, but then, well, people'd wind him up as well.

'Yeah, but, weird this, I mean, people do wind me up when I've been drinking. And, well, I mean, I dunno, sometimes I feel like I'd like it to be different.'

'Different?'

'I don't know, there's always some arsehole in your face. Sometimes, I don't know, I want to get away from all that.'

'Get away from arseholes in your face, you mean?'

'Yeah, I mean, yeah. In the town, you know, it gets pretty crazy, I mean the bars are really full, music's loud, and that's, yeah, that's OK, and there's a few laughs, you know. But sometimes I just feel like I want to get away. I don't say nothing, well, I mean, you don't. But sometimes, yeah, sometimes I just want to get away.'

'Away from the packed bars and everything?'

Gary nodded. 'But what do you do, where do you go? And, I mean, I don't imagine my mates would be interested.'

'So, feeling like you want to get away but where to, and would your mates want that?'

Gary took a deep breath. 'I get tired of it all, sometimes. I really do. Just want to be left alone, people out of my space.'

'Get away, people out of your space, something different, huh?'

'Yeah ...' Gary paused. 'Yeah, something different.'

The idea of a something else, of a quiet drink without hassle has been present for Gary before in the counselling sessions. He is now more responsive to that urge. He is talking about it more freely, more open to the idea, although he can't at the moment imagine how it could happen. He is not denying the possibility of what he is desiring; the yearning is present in Gary's awareness and is being held there. This is a change. The counsellor stays with the client, offering careful empathy, enabling Gary to explore more of what he is experiencing, allowing him to encounter and engage with this aspect of himself.

'Mhmm.' Rick left Gary with what he was thinking about. He sensed that Gary was thinking about what 'something different' meant to him. Rick was aware that they were words he had used, that he had introduced, and yet they felt as though they captured the gist of what Gary had been saying, and maybe they were reflecting what was present for Gary even though he hadn't expressed it quite that way. He waited for Gary to speak.

'I'm tired of getting wound up, and ending up at hospital, stuff like that. Yeah, it's a laugh as well, but it gets to me too.'

'Gets to you?'

'Be good to go out and come home, just that, you know? Just come home feeling, yeah, feeling relaxed. I mean a few beers, yeah, they relax me, but, I don't know, I'm never relaxed at the end of the evening, always wound up, always something happens, you know? Always end up feeling so fucking angry.'

'Something about when you go out, the things that happen leave you feeling angry and you don't want that?'

'I don't. I wish I wasn't, you know? I wish I could relax a bit more.'

'Finding a way to be relaxed just sounds so important to you.'

Gary took a deep breath and relaxed his shoulders. His back was tight. But he didn't stretch too much, he knew it would set his ribs off. 'And I get fed up being in pain, you know? Always something. I just want a bit of a quiet life. I mean, I don't want to not go out and drink and stuff, don't get me wrong, I just wish it was different.'

'Mhmm, don't want to give up going out, having a few drinks, just want it to be a, what, different kind of experience?'

'Yeah, yeah, but everywhere's so in your face. And, yeah, I'm up for that as well, but sometimes . . .' He took another deep breath and let it out slowly. 'You know?'

'Yeah, sometimes . . . , not so much in your face.' Rick was aware that the pace of the session seemed to have slowed. Not that it had been fast, it was probably something subjective, how he was feeling. It felt appropriate though, an aspect of what seemed a more reflective state, and he wondered briefly whether Gary was feeling the same way. 'I have a sense of something to do with slowing down.'

> Rick is sharing his genuinely felt experience from the context of feeling integrated in the relationship. He is owning the experience, not trying to tell the client how it is. It is tentative, an offering of what has become present for him. It's like an experience that might be described as, 'hey, I feel we're connecting here, and this is emerging for me, how about you?'.

Gary thought about it. 'Yeah, yeah, something like that. Slow down, yeah. Yeah.'

'Mhmm.'

Gary thought about it. 'Yeah, that's what I need. Take it easy, that's OK, take it easy. Have to anyway at the moment with my ribs.'

'Yeah, they've slowed you down.'

For some reason Gary's thoughts were back with why he'd been referred to the counselling in the first place, his GP thinking he drank too much. The thought was in Gary's head that, yeah, drinking did sort of get him into trouble. But it wasn't that his drinking was a problem, just that trouble happened. It confused him a bit, and he didn't like people telling him what was or wasn't good for him. People on his case, yeah, that wound him up. He wished people would let him alone, let him get on with his life. Not that he knew much about what he wanted, live day to day, week to week. Work, get some dosh in your pocket, go out, have a good time, get drunk, screw around, yeah, and not have the hassle. Why did he always end up in trouble? Why? The question seemed very present to him as he sat there.

> The client experiences confusion as he begins to accept the notion that his drinking gets him into trouble. The part of him that likes/needs the

> excitement and the release of alcohol-fuelled violence and aggression, and the part of him that wants to slow down are both very present in the client's awareness. The result is a fundamental conflict, two competing needs, and as a result anxiety will arise. In a sense he wants both and behind what is present is his ongoing need to ensure that he does not allow the idea that he is in any way like his father to break into his awareness and threaten his self-concept.

Rick sat with the silence that had emerged between them once again. It didn't feel awkward, as though Gary didn't know what to say. He sort of seemed lost in his own thoughts again. 'Lot to think about, huh.'

'Hmm? Yeah, yeah, sort of, I don't know, kind of wondering why I always seem to end up with trouble, you know? Why?'

'Why you, you mean?'

Gary nodded. 'Yeah, things happen, you know?'

'Things . . . ?'

'People, in my space, sad bastards that just, yeah, like I've said before, in your face, arseholes, can't hold their drink, they piss me off.'

'Arseholes who can't hold their drink, they really piss you off.' Rick stayed with Gary's language, keeping his empathic response focused not just on what was being said, but also the way it was being communicated.

Gary was shaking his head and Rick could see that his body was tensing up again. 'Winds you up, just thinking about it.'

'Yeah, it does. And, yeah, it's like part of me just doesn't want it, doesn't want the hassle, yeah? And then, well, yeah, I also want to get in there and sort it.' He was nodding now. 'Yeah, that's how it is. I don't apologise to no one.'

Rick was struck by the last comment. It had sort of emerged from nowhere as far as he was concerned. He responded, being brief, not wanting to disrupt what had emerged and where it might lead. 'Don't apologise to no one.'

Gary thought. 'No, I mean, you know, if it's a mate, I mean, yeah, well, sometimes.'

'Even if it's a mate then sometimes you will, sometimes not?'

'Depends. Usually depends on how pissed I am!' Gary grinned.

Rick returned the smile. 'So what you're saying is that you're less likely to apologise, even to mates, when you're pissed?'

'I guess so. Yeah, I guess that's how it is.'

'Mhmm. OK. That's how it is. Less likely to apologise when you're pissed.'

'And more likely to get wound up as well, yeah?'

'When you're pissed you get more wound up. Kind of gets to you more.'

Gary nodded. 'I get more angry, irritated, yeah, people piss me off.'

'Yeah, you get pissed and people piss you off, yeah?'

'Yeah.' The tone of voice had become sharper, Gary was bringing some feelings into what he was saying.

Rick nodded. 'And the more pissed you are, the more pissed off you get?'

Gary thought for a moment. 'Yeah, sort of, probably, I'll lash out more, yeah, that's what my mates say, I'll react more when I'm pissed, pile in, you know, get in there.'

'OK, so when you're pissed and people are more likely to piss you off, you're more likely to pile in, yeah?'

'Yeah.' Gary was feeling tense. He was thinking back to an incident in a bar not long back where some guy with a loud voice had kept bumping into him, well, twice, but that was enough. He'd reacted. Given him some verbal. The guy'd backed down, but if he hadn't, Gary knew he was ready to have a go at him. Even now, thinking about it, he could feel himself tensing up. 'Yeah. I mean, you've got to, haven't you?'

'It sounds like *you've* got to?'

'Well, yeah. Yeah, I do. I mean, I don't like, you know, people just . . ., they craze you, you know?'

'Craze you? Not sure I understand exactly what you're meaning.'

'Get to you. I mean, you go out, have a few beers, few laughs, but someone's always, I don't know, someone's looking at you, or spills drink on you, or knocks into you, and I don't like it. Don't want it, you know?'

'Mhmm.'

Gary was shaking his head. People giving him grief, yeah . . .

The session continued with Gary not really adding a great deal more to what he had already being saying, while remaining sure in himself that it was a matter of it being everyone else's problem, not his. He just tried to sort things out, sort people out, who 'crazed him'. He wasn't thinking or feeling that his drinking, or his past, had anything to do with his sensitivity, his rather reactive and volatile nature after 'a few beers', as he liked to describe it.

The session ended and Gary left. He felt troubled. He wasn't sure why, a sort of unease, something didn't feel right inside himself. He knew he felt like a drink, that would settle him back down. Maybe he'd go out, he'd give his mates a ring and organise something. Felt like he needed to get off his face, what the hell, and if someone upset him, tough on them. He took a kick at a can on the path, yeah, fuck his ribs, he was going to enjoy himself tonight.

Rick, meanwhile, was sitting back in his chair pondering on the session. So much irritation in Gary, so much pissed him off, he was so caught up in sorting people, situations out, and so clear that he wasn't like his father. That sense of him needing to know that he wasn't an 'alcy'. The nurse must have got to him. Interesting. It wasn't that he'd blanked it or forgotten about it, clearly she'd made an impression, but Gary wasn't going to believe her, and yet he wasn't able to let go of it either. He started to write his notes, wondering how or when Gary might make a connection between his past, his drinking and his reactions to people and situations. They were clearly emerging, but would Gary be able to stay open to them, or would he need to shut them down, maybe using more alcohol to block out the discrepancy between his self-concept and what might break into his awareness? There was, of course, no point in pushing it. Gary would see it as and when it became clear to him.

Or maybe circumstances would make it clear, or something. And besides, too much material breaking into awareness and threatening a person's self-concept could be a shattering experience, and one that needed to occur at a pace dictated by the client.

As a person-centred counsellor Rick was clear that his role was to convey his empathic understanding and warmly accept Gary as he was, as he needed to be, as he experienced himself. Gary was the way he was for reasons rooted in the way he had developed his concept of self in reaction to his life experiences. He'd been brought up in an unpredictable and threatening environment. Boundaries were probably very unclear. There may not have been much consistent loving. There was threat in the air and actual violence. It would all have made an impression, and in the midst a young boy had been trying to find a sense of identity, learn how to be, what was acceptable, what enabled him to get his needs met.

Now, it seemed, his need was to release anger and frustration, to lash out, to not tolerate anything or anyone that made him feel a certain way – 'pissed off', 'crazed'. Rick trusted himself to be able to consistently offer the therapeutic conditions. He did not know how big an impact this would have or was having on Gary, but he trusted that it would be making an impression and that he needed to maintain his way of being, so that perhaps, in time, Gary might begin to be more open to possibilities about himself that he was clearly closed to at present. But for that to occur he would need to feel safe enough to risk confronting the fact that perhaps, to some degree, he was evidencing some of the traits of his father, the man, the 'alcy' that represented a set of behaviours that had become symbolised in his awareness as something he must never be or become.

Points for discussion

- What are your thoughts and feelings towards Gary as a person? Does this differ in any way to how you might previously have felt about a young person drinking and fighting?
- What particular qualities of person-centred practice did Rick evidence in this last session?
- What aspects of Gary's self-concept do you see as being directly linked to his past?
- Were there any key moments in the session? What is it that contributes to a moment being key or particularly significant in the therapeutic process?
- What would you take to supervision from this session?

Write notes for the session.

CHAPTER 4

Counselling session 5: more from the past and an uneasy insight

Wednesday 14 May

'Been a bit edgy this week, never really got settled. Bad week, I guess, everyone has them.'

'Bad week for you, edgy, not settled.'

'People in your face, messing you about. Work was crap. Dunno, just wasn't interested, you know?'

'Mhmm.' Rick nodded, sensing the strength of irritation in Gary's voice. It sounded like he really was fed up with how his week had been

'Yeah, drank a bit too much as well, probably. Had a few heavy nights, you know?' He forced a grin. Rick smiled back.

'So, not a good week for your drinking, then?'

'Too much, yeah, suppose I overdid it, had a good time though. Went for it last week, after being here. Just needed a drink, needed to get out and get lashed.' He shrugged, thinking back to what he could remember of the events of last Wednesday. It was still a bit hazy. They'd all three of them gone out and, well, they were still drinking well into the early hours. And, yeah, there had been a couple of 'arguments', nothing he hadn't been able to handle, on one occasion he'd had to threaten to knock some sense into someone who was getting on his nerves. They'd backed down.

'So, you felt after the last session here that you needed to really down a few, yeah?'

'Don't know why, just did. It's like that sometimes.'

'Sometimes you mean it sort of feels different, like you just sort of have to really, as you say, go out and get lashed?'

'I guess I was wound up, you know, what we'd been talking about and stuff. Things you think about, you know, get to you, does my head in sometimes. A few drinks, helps me settle, but this week, well, it hasn't. I just feel fuckin' awful.' Gary still knew he didn't feel on top form, he'd had a heavy drinking weekend as well. Hadn't felt good but, well, thought it'd make him feel better.

Now, a week later, he was still feeling edgy, still couldn't feel comfortable. He just felt generally fed up. He got like this sometimes. Lost interest in things. Everything seemed too much effort. He was a bit like that anyway.

'So, this week, the drinking hasn't helped, in fact you're left feeling awful, yeah?'

Gary didn't respond. His thoughts had drifted back into his childhood again. He hadn't really thought about it this way, but he had spent more time that last week thinking about his past, and feeling stuff towards his father. He wasn't making any conscious link between this and his drinking, it had simply become a focus for his thinking more than usual.

Rick had another thought that had intruded into his awareness, resulting from a TV programme he had watched recently, about how diet seemed to affect the mood of young people, particularly junk food. The sugar, the fat, the lack of natural vitamins and minerals where a young person's diet was 'burger-and-chips centred'. It had made an impression on him and it seemed that there was increasing evidence that for many young people, some of the 'syndromes' that they were being diagnosed with might actually be less a mental health issue and more a nutritional problem. He brought his thinking back to Gary, and to the way that Gary saw his awful week as being linked to overdoing it with the drinking. That was Gary's reality; that was the way he was experiencing himself, and that was what Rick was there to communicate empathic under-standing of.

> Thoughts do intrude on a counsellor's concentration on their client, and sometimes the thoughts emerge because they are particularly pressing for the therapist – and therefore need dealing with, in supervision and/or ther-apy – and sometimes they may have relevance to what the client is expres-sing or revealing. In the latter case the therapist needs to decide whether what has come into their awareness is emerging in the context of the ther-apeutic relationship, or not. Often, such thoughts, if they are emerging from the therapeutic relationship, will do so when there is a particular sense of connection with the client. In the above instance, this does not seem to be the case. This does not mean that what he is thinking about does not have relevance for the client, but it is not what we might term a 'therapeutically emergent insight'.

'I wish I could stop thinking about memories, you know? I mean, it's past, I want to move on but then, well, I sort of don't, it's like, yeah, it's part of me, you know? It's my history and, yeah, I sort of need to respect that in some way.'

'Like you need to respect it because it's sort of part of you, part of your story, so to speak?'

Gary nodded, and he also noted a sense of wishing it wasn't part of his story as well. But he couldn't imagine how different his life could be. Yeah, he saw some of the programmes on TV, the American families, all friendly and stuff. But it was unreal – unreal to him. That wasn't how life was, and he knew he wasn't alone, some of his mates had had tough times as well. And it had made him toughen up, he reckoned. Yeah, he wouldn't take any shit from anyone, not now, not now he could fight back. He hated thinking about not being able to fight back, like it had been when he was a kid. Now, well, now he fought back first, get it sorted.

'I don't take shit from anyone.' He looked at Rick as he spoke, it was more of a stare. Rick sensed the challenge in his eyes. He nodded as he responded.

'Mhmm, you don't take shit ... , from *anyone*.' He spoke slowly and sought to respond with the same emphasis that he had heard in Gary's voice.

Gary continued to stare. He was in another place. Not a very psychological way of describing it, but that was his reality. He got into that state of mind, a sort of determination to fight, to not take anything from anyone that he didn't want to hear, or experience. It was a strong place. It was a place where Gary felt good, whole, focused, intense. He liked to feel that way. He didn't often think of it like that, but that was how it was. It gave him a good sense of self, of satisfaction.

Rick sat with his sense of what Gary was communicating through his eyes and his whole demeanour, and aware of his own response. Here was a young man with attitude, no mistaking that, and powerful attitude at that. He could well imagine that Gary must feel good feeling how he did when he was like this. He sensed that there was a power present. He accepted it. He didn't fear it, simply acknowledged its presence. Yes, it did impact on him, of course it did. But he felt a warmth, given his understanding of some of the experiences Gary had had.

'Feels powerful, does to me hearing you speak, being here with you.'

Gary nodded. He suddenly moved his head and broke the eye contact. 'Yeah. I get like that, you know, that's me.' He shrugged.

'Mhmm, how you can be, some of the time.' Rick wanted to acknowledge that he had heard both that it was how Gary could be, but also that it was how he was some of the time, not all of the time.

Gary suddenly swallowed, he felt strange, his stomach churned, he felt unsettled, anxious, he didn't know what it was. It was different from how he usually felt. There was a sadness, and then it was gone. He screwed his eyes tight for a moment. The sensations remained but were easing. He took a deep breath, not sure what to make of it, and decided not to try.

> This could be more material emerging from the edge of his awareness, but it has been fleeting, not strong or persistent enough to remain in his awareness. It can be disorientating for the client who may be suddenly filled with feelings that he has no rational explanation for.

Rick saw Gary screw his eyes up but had no sense of why. The room felt quiet and yet there seemed to be an intensity in the atmosphere. Was that where it was, or was it simply within his own inner world and he projected it out on to the room, the space around him? He noticed Gary move in the chair; he was moving his shoulders, he guessed he must be feeling stiff.

'I keep thinking about the past, more since I've been coming here. I don't like it, but can't sort of stop it.' Gary was shaking his head again. 'I mean, yeah, it was tough, wasn't good, but, well, I s'ppose it was OK as well, I mean, didn't do me any harm. Just how it was, not like those TV shows, all happy families. Well, those American ones anyway. You see more reality on British TV, yeah, kids from hell and all that stuff, yeah, don't often see parents from hell though, do you? Well, no, I mean, mum was OK, she was good, did her best, but ...' He shook his head, thinking again of his father. 'Why did I have to have such a bastard for a father?' He was shaking his head again. 'Why couldn't he, I don't know, not been such a fucking ...' again he shook his head. He wasn't sure he knew quite what to say. He hated him for how he'd been. Made him feel angry. He could feel himself tightening and tensing up.

Rick saw the tension in Gary, and the hardness in his face. 'Why couldn't he have been ... different?'

Gary nodded. 'Yeah, OK, I wouldn't want him to be all sort of, I don't know, I wanted someone I could look up to, you know?'

Rick nodded, aware that there was something suddenly different in the way Gary was speaking. There was a clear ownership of what he had wanted, and it suddenly felt really important that his response conveyed that he both heard and felt warmth for what Gary was saying and experiencing – a son wanting a father he could look up to.

'Yeah, a father to look up to, feel proud of, have respect for ...' Rick knew his response was more comprehensive than what Gary had said, but the words had just formed as he had begun speaking. Maybe it was partly his own stuff, what he had felt important in his own life, but also informed by the way Gary had been speaking.

'Yeah, respect for ...' Gary shook his head.

Damn, though Rick, I shouldn't have used that word, it's shifted Gary away from what he wanted into what was lacking.

The counsellor has justified his response to Gary, but the reality is that it was too clever, trying to bring in words that at that moment were not those that were present for Gary. The counsellor has unwittingly directed the client's focus away in the way that Rick has now realised. He tries to re-establish the focus.

'You just wanted someone to look up to.'

'It's not much to ask, is it? Instead, I get an alcy for a father who beats up my mother and pisses off.' He shook his head again. 'I never want to be like that. If I get married, have kids, I'll never be like that. I wouldn't want my kids to go through what I did.'

To Rick, Gary seemed almost reflective as he spoke. He empathised. 'You wouldn't want to put them through what you experienced.'

'No.' He took a deep breath. 'No.' The unease returned again. He sniffed, he had a
 tissue somewhere. He checked his pockets, found it and blew his nose.

He didn't know why he said it, but he heard the words coming out of his mouth.
 They seemed strangely distant, but it was his voice. 'I've fucked up, haven't I?'

'That how it feels, you've fucked up?'

'Yeah. I lose it, don't I?'

'What in particular?'

'Everything.'

'That bad?'

Gary felt quiet, although the unease was there as well. He felt slightly sick. And
 his hands and arms had a strange sort of tingly numbness, he didn't know how
 else to think of it.

'Yeah, I mean, yeah, have a few laughs, but, shit, yeah, I've fucked up.'

Rick didn't know why Gary was suddenly speaking like this, but it felt very present and powerful, and important for him to be very accurate in his responses.
 He didn't know where it would go but he trusted that what was happening was
 timely for Gary, and he knew he shouldn't say or do anything that might get in
 the way. Gary was telling him that he'd fucked up – he hadn't really described
 exactly what he meant, but clearly he, Gary, knew what he meant.

'You mean sort of you have a few laughs. But, you feel like you've fucked up.'

'I don't know. Gets you down. I mean, yeah, Like going out, doing stuff, yeah,
 course I do. But like I've said before, I kind of get tired of it as well. Sometimes,
 yeah, sometimes I want a quiet life as well. And, yeah, I think of my old man, I
 mean ...' Gary shook his head as he thought about him, how he had been,
 what he meant to him now, 'what a sad bastard'.

Rick noted the word 'sad', not a word he'd heard Gary use in relation to his father
 before.

'Sad bastard?'

'Well, I mean, he fucked up, didn't he.' Gary went quiet. Rick waited, only too
 aware of what Gary had just said and what he had been saying a little while
 before. What connection was Gary making, and to what effect?

Gary was taking a deep breath, somehow he didn't know what to say or feel, he
 felt shocked and very quiet. He was shaking his head slightly and could feel
 words forming his head. 'I'm not like him, I can't be, I'm different. He lost it,
 I'm OK, I'm in control.' The words were internal, his mouth and jaw were
 firmly set. In the midst of his sudden numbness he could feel that anxiety,
 unease again. And a kind of sick feeling in his stomach. But he wasn't like
 him, he wasn't, course he wasn't. Yeah, he got into fights, but that was different, people got in his face, arseholes who deserved to be sorted. He didn't
 go looking for trouble ... , but he had to admit that it usually found him, or
 he found it. He looked up. He still felt a strange creeping numbness in his
 body, his arms and sort of in his head, and yet he suddenly felt so alert, but
 that unease, he felt really strange. It felt as though he was sort of spaced out,
 bit like being drunk but not really, similar but different. Didn't feel right to
 feel like this and be stone cold sober. He felt confused, and wasn't sure what
 to say.

Rick had noticed Gary look up and had caught his eye. He felt the stillness and the intensity as well, and also felt unsure what to say. It didn't seem right to break the silence, somehow that silence was, well, strange thing to think, but it was a very loud silence. Deafening in a way, but that wasn't quite the right way to describe it. Just very intense. He realised he was frowning, feeling a tension in his own face. It was partly as a result of his concentration, and maybe he was also in some way physically paralleling Gary, who he realised was also frowning with what seemed an expression of puzzlement on his face as well. The silence continued.

Gary swallowed, still looking at Rick, and then looked away. He felt that sadness again. Again words came to him and he heard himself speaking them. They were his words, and yet there was a strange distance between him and them, but they were close as well, so much part of him. 'Why did he have to be like he was?'

Rick felt himself taking a deep breath as he heard Gary speak. It was as though his body was reacting, needing to take on more oxygen, more life, more energy. The words hung in the air, and they needed a response. They demanded a response.

'Why?' Rick spoke quietly and reflectively, seeking to convey his hearing of Gary but seeking to ensure his minimal response did not intrude on Gary's focus.

Gary was shaking his head. 'I hated him so much, for how he was. I was ashamed of him. Other kids would laugh but I was ashamed. I'd get angry, lash out. I hated it, hate them, hated him.' It was Gary's turn to take a deep breath.

'Hated them, hated him, hated it all.'

The sadness was more present for Gary and he could feel his eyes watering, but he wasn't going to let Rick see. He widened them to try to absorb back the tears in some way. 'They taunted me, bastards. Sometimes it was OK . . .' He shook his head. 'But usually it wasn't. I'd be angry. I had to control it, sometimes I could, but not always. Close mates were OK, you know, they sort of understood, they were OK, yeah, real mates, like Mal and Luke, they've known me for a long time, been together through tough times. Not been easy for them either, but they, well, I don't know, they didn't have to face what I had to face. But somehow they stuck with me. Good mates, you know?' He looked up again and looked into Rick's eyes.

'Yeah good, mates, we all need them.' He felt his own eyes watering as well. It felt very powerful, somehow in the moment the two of them were meeting in some way that was deeper, two people united by a common recognition of the need to have good mates. Rick knew the truth of that from his own experience, yet he also knew he was there to listen to what Gary had to say.

Gary sensed that Rick understood, not by what he said, but how he had said it and how he looked. It felt important. 'Yeah.'

There seemed to be a moment of mutual understanding, both of them in their own way acknowledging how important good mates were; for Gary it sort of made Rick seem more real somehow. Not that he had felt unreal to him, but it was like it was something they were really agreeing on. It wasn't that it felt enormously significant, but it was there, a sense, an experience. Gary sort of felt a little more at ease.

It was Gary who spoke first after the silence that arose between them. 'I guess I wish things had been different, and I guess, well, yeah, I suppose I sort of know that, well, how things were, you know, sort of affected me.'

Rick nodded, aware that what Gary had said had sounded sort of hesitant and yet there was a clear recognition behind those words. He responded with a little more focus. 'You wish things had been different and, yeah, you can see that it affected you.'

'He was a bastard.' Gary was looking directly at Rick, who returned the eye contact.

'Mhmm.' Rick nodded slightly as he responded, not feeling that there was much to really say in response, other than an acknowledgement that he was listening.

Gary was shaking his head. 'He just couldn't cope, I don't know why, and just drank, and got bitter, and violent, and, well, took it out on mum mostly. He'd have a go at me sometimes as well. Maybe that's why I react now. Maybe it's because of him, you know? I mean, I couldn't do anything then, I couldn't. Just had to keep out of his way. Can't do that now. Don't want to do that. I'm not going to be like that, I fight, stand my ground, don't take nothing from no one, know what I mean?'

'Mmm, like you can't afford to be like you were . . .'

'. . . no, I'm not going to let anyone push me around.' Gary was shaking his head. 'But I guess I, well, Mal and Luke think I over-react sometimes. They seem to be able to be in control. Yeah, they'll fight, but they seem more controlled, not like me. I sort of lose it. Things become personal, you know?' He shrugged. 'I have to sort it.'

'It feels personal for you and it's important for you to sort it.'

'Two things.' Gary was nodding as he spoke. 'Two things: I'm not going to get like my old man, and I'm not going to let anyone push me around. That's how it is, how I have to be. How I want to be, I guess. I mean, yeah, don't take shit from anyone.'

'Mhmm, sounds pretty clear, don't be like your old man and take no shit from anyone. Feels like how you have to be.'

'Yeah . . . yeah, that's me. And mostly it's OK, I can handle it, you know, but there are times I just want, you know, like I've said, to have less hassle. I just lose it though. Few drinks, bevvied up and then, bang, I go. I'll pick a fight with anyone, anyone, anything that upsets me, gets in my space, in my face, and I'm there. I can feel it now, talking about it. I tense up and then . . .' he paused. 'That's me.'

'That's you, get bevvied up, something upsets you and bang, you're in there.'

The client has moved into a more reflective place. He can see how he is. He is not so strongly identifying with it, but can observe it as a part of his nature. He has previously engaged with strong feelings, feelings of sadness, the hate towards those who taunted him, his appreciation of having good mates. In fact, it has been a very powerful phase in the session for Gary. He has allowed himself to feel and communicate those feelings within the therapy session, feelings that are not always those that he might make visible to others or to himself. The person-centred counsellor seeks to accept all that Gary is experiencing and perceiving about himself. What is being revealed are important aspects of Gary's inner world, both now and in the past.

His childhood experiences encouraged him to develop particular ways of thinking about himself and how he needed to be. Feeling threatened and powerless in the presence of his drunk and violent father caused him to vow never to be like him, and never to allow himself to be a victim in the way that he was forced to be in the past. He reacts by refusing to allow himself to think of himself as weak. He has to be strong, he has to stand up, fight back. He internalises the need to be that way. It will satisfy his need to not feel victimised, to not feel powerless. As a result he develops a sense of self, or self-concept, that he is strong, doesn't take shit from anyone, and to prove it he has to behave in a certain way, which he does, reinforcing and maintaining his self-concept.

The difficulty for Gary is that he also has vowed never to be like his father. Any behaviour that might on the face of it seem to be like his father cannot be seen that way by Gary. So his alcohol use has to have a different meaning to him, has to be seen as somehow not the same as his father's drinking. He cannot possibly accept any notion that he might be behaving like his father. He defends himself by describing his father as an 'alcy', something that he is not because, perhaps, he doesn't drink in settings like his father did, or does. And he knows he wouldn't be like his father, violent towards a woman, or children.

'I mean, yeah, people wind me up. I mean, that's why it happens. They get under my skin, you know? Not like my old man, he was just . . ., he'd just come home and, well, anything, any reason at all and he'd go for us, but mainly mum. Over nothing, he'd react, you know? Fucking nutter. That's what he was, he really, was – well, still is, not that I see him much. He's maybe quietened down now, don't think he gets violent now, I don't know, I don't care.' There was a tinge of sadness, but Gary's feelings were mixed. Yes, he did feel sad, but he was angry too, and the anger was more powerful. But the sadness was there. He found it hard to admit to, though. He didn't want to feel sympathy for his old man. He was bad news, had made his life, both their lives, a bloody misery and he was glad he wasn't around.

'Yeah, people wind you up, but it seems different from how you experienced your father.'

'He'd blow up about nothing, anything. Just a fucking nonsense. Just tried to keep out of his way. You could never get anything right, whatever you did was wrong.' Gary took a deep breath. He couldn't make sense of it, had given up trying. 'Shit life. Fuck him. I just don't want to be like him.'

'Don't want to be like him, and it feels more like "mustn't be like him".'

'Yeah,' Gary was shaking his head again. It felt good to talk. He'd never ever talked like this in his life, not like this, not sober, and not to someone who sort of didn't judge him, just listened, paid attention. Weird, but not weird. It felt good. He couldn't make sense of it, just felt like he needed to talk and, yeah, Rick seemed to listen, to understand. Didn't try to make him think anything, didn't question him – yeah, he didn't want that, someone poking their nose into his business. Rick didn't do that. Seemed to Gary that he sort of just sat and listened, said what he heard, accepted what he heard. Yeah, felt easier somehow, easier than when he'd talked about his drinking.

He noticed the time, it was almost the end of the session. He sort of didn't want to go. It felt strange but it felt good to be just sitting like this. Wasn't something he'd imagined himself thinking, or feeling, but that was how it was. Just felt like he wanted to be quiet. 'Thanks.'

'Thanks?'

'For listening. Helped me get a few things off my chest. Few things to think about as well. I need to head off. I just need to get stuff out of my head, you know?'

Rick nodded, aware of his own sense of the intensity that he could hear in Gary's voice, intense and yet there was what seemed like a tiredness as well. He wasn't surprised. As the session drew to a close he found himself wondering how different Gary's life had been to his own. He'd not had the kind of experiences that Gary had been subject to, and the effects, well, he heard them from his clients. Gary had to be not like his father. And yet, he had to drink to cope, release pent-up feelings and use aggression to deal with situations, some of which he probably provoked or looked for as a reason to be how he needed to be. And that was it, Gary was being how he needed to be. He had to let his self-concept find expression, he had to be himself. But it was a sense of self rooted in powerful, conditioning experiences.

For Rick, the challenge and the opportunity of being a person-centred therapist was to enable his clients to gain a fresh sense of self within the experience of a relationship in which they felt warmly accepted, where there was a clear attempt being made for them to be heard and understood, where there was an openness, a transparency, an authenticity present in the therapist, offering opportunity for this to become more present for the client within the relationship. He knew that when people began to redefine themselves emotionally and psychologically, when they began to grow into or develop a fresh sense of self through the quality and nature of the therapeutic experience, constructive personality change could and would occur. But unlike other more directive therapies, or where there is a stronger sense of the counsellor knowing what intervention would be best for the client or what the client needed to focus on, he trusted that the actualising tendency within the client would operate through the therapeutic relational experience to bring about an opportunity for the client to re-assess himself – not necessarily in a cognitive way, but at a more visceral level, where so often the real difficulties existed and which drove the client to think about himself in particular ways.

Five minutes later and Gary was heading for work. He didn't understand how he felt. It was confusing. He felt sort of calm, somehow, that intense churning unease had passed, so had the anger, and yet ... He could sense that they were not far away, still very much part of him. He had been surprised at what he had said, and the way he had spoken to Rick. He didn't understand this counselling. And yet it somehow felt good, even though he couldn't really explain what was happening to him. His thoughts were back with his father, and his mother as well, and how difficult it had been for her to bring him up. But she had. Yes, he'd had problems, and still did, and maybe always would, but somehow he sort of knew he needed to be different, to change. He liked the buzz, the excitement of going out, but he knew he was getting tired of the fights, tired of getting angry. Yes, that was it, tired of getting angry – with other people, with his father and, well, he sort of felt angry with himself for getting angry as well. That seemed a bit weird.

He was so deep in thought that he missed the turning he needed to take. Found himself going down a road he hadn't been down before. Well, it wasn't too much of a detour, and actually it sort of made a change. He didn't think about it much more, but at some level or place in himself there was an experience of feeling good about going a different way. It was outside his awareness, over the edge of his horizon, as it were.

Points for discussion

- What thoughts and feelings are you left with from this session? How does Gary affect you? What does he bring of you into your awareness?
- What were the significant features of this counselling session?
- When might you, as the counsellor, have responded differently, and why?
- How would you describe the therapeutic relationship, avoiding the use of psycho-jargon?
- How effective was Rick in offering empathy and unconditional positive regard, and maintaining his own congruence?
- What might you take to supervision from this session?

Write notes for the session.

CHAPTER 5

Supervision session 2: to reflect on the process of material from edge of awareness and self-concept under threat

Friday 16 May

'I want to explore my work with Gary, Jean, and in particular the impact on him, and on me, of material emerging from, well, let's say from the edge of his awareness. In fact I think it's more from over the edge of his awareness.'

'More over the edge?' Jean's response was questioning; she appreciated what Rick was saying, but was curious to hear what Gary's experience was.

'Ideas, notions, thoughts about himself, things that he's denied to awareness – and I'm tempted to say consciously or unconsciously here though quite what I mean by that I am unsure.'

'As if what you are saying isn't clear to you?'

'I don't know how you can unconsciously deny something to awareness. I can see that you might be unaware that something is not being allowed into conscious awareness, but that feels different. It's hard to define somehow.' Rick frowned as he thought about what he had said. He felt he wanted to use different words, conscious/unconscious didn't feel right, somehow.

'So it is something about whether there is an unconscious process?'

Rick nodded. 'It's not a way of thinking that comes naturally to me. Who I am is a product of my experiences and how I have symbolised them in awareness. This leads me to develop a concept of who I am. And, well, yeah, the me that I am, that I experience myself as being, is made up of things that are, well, truly me, and things that I've taken on board from others. I work towards fuller congruence, but it's like there is incongruence in the system, parts of me that react or respond to situations that I've learned. Following somebody else's pattern. I feel like I've addressed a lot over the years, working on myself, trying to be fully and openly aware to what is being experienced, and being able to be accurate in my understanding of myself.'

Rogers has defined congruence as being: 'When self-experiences are accurately symbolized and are included in the self-concept in this accurately symbolized form, then the state is one of congruence of self and experience' (Rogers, 1959, p.206). By contrast, he defines incongruence in the following terms: 'It refers to a discrepancy between the actual experience of the organism and the self picture of the individual as it represents that experience' (Rogers, 1957a, p.96). Gary has symbolised aggression within his self-concept. It is OK to be aggressive. In reality his alcohol-fuelled aggression means he is behaving like his father, but he cannot allow this recognition to be made, for it would threaten his self-concept which sees his anger and aggression as positive aspects of his nature, of his ability to sort things out, to feel strong. He must not let himself see himself as being like his father although in reality he is, and as a result of his denying this there is a discrepancy between his experience and his self-picture. And therefore he is in an incongruent state and anxiety will be present, and more so if the realisation that he is like his father enters his awareness.

As can often be the case, the alcohol use may be partly to help push away this awareness, although in fact it actually encourages the behaviour that reinforces it. This is not unusual where substances are involved to affect awareness.

Jean nodded. 'OK, so you can see how you have worked on yourself to gain greater congruence, greater accuracy in your awareness of your experiencing . . .'

Rick interrupted her. '. . . yes, yes, but for Gary, I mean, he doesn't have this insight, and in a way I want to say he's protected or protecting himself from it. There is no doubt that while he says to me, as he has, that he mustn't be "like his father", the reality is that he is being. And when that really makes an impact on his awareness, it really is going to throw him. And I suspect it is happening and I am concerned that it will cause him to spin off into heavier drinking to cope, and with that will come added anger and frustration associated with what he has glimpsed about himself. It really feels like this is a critical time for Gary. Things are moving to the surface. The way he is, the way he is speaking. He is becoming more self-reflective and, I don't know, it's going to dawn on him. I mean, he knows he gets violent and aggressive, he knows he drinks heavily, but he still sees it as different. Maybe he'll be able to preserve this for a while. I don't know. But I don't think so. And that's because he seems more reflective. It's like . . .' Rick paused, unsure how to express himself.

'His being more reflective . . . ?'

Rick pursed his lips and took a deep breath. 'Last session he was quite critical and condemning of his father. Said that his father had fucked up, but also said he'd fucked up as well. And there was a period of silence, a really intense silence in that session. And he talked sort of differently for a short while afterwards, asking why his father had had to be like that. And how he had hated him and the other kids that used to taunt him because of his father. Then the session moved away from that, I think he got into saying how he couldn't be like his father.' Rick was aware that he was frowning as he spoke. He was concentrating, somehow that part of the session had felt important even though he did not know what Gary was really thinking or feeling.

'So he hated his father.'

'For being alcy and for being violent towards his mother, and himself. He talked of having to keep out of the way. Quite how abusive his father was to him I don't know, but it seems likely that he was physically abusive, and he clearly witnessed how his father was towards his mother.'

Jean nodded, wondering how long it had been like that for Gary. Had he known anything different in childhood? It was one thing when a child had experienced feeling loved by parents and then had to cope with abusive behaviour, but something else when that abuse had been present from those very early formative years. 'And we don't know for how long, how early it started?'

'I don't think so, I'm not sure, but I kind of . . . , no, I don't know, or at least if I do I can't recall.'

'I'm just thinking about how fragile he might be, thinking about how children not receiving empathic understanding, something I remember reading about "fragile process".'

The idea is that clients who as children experienced 'empathic failure' go on to 'experience a "fragile" style of processing as adults . . . Clients who have a fragile style of processing tend to experience core issues at very high or low levels of intensity. They tend to have difficulty starting and stopping experiences that are personally significant or emotionally connected' (Warner, 2000, p.150; see also Warner 1991, 1997). Elsewhere Warner writes that 'because they have difficulty holding on to their own experience, they often have difficulty taking in the point of view of another person without feeling that their own experience has been annihilated', and she gives the following example: '. . . a client may talk in a low-key way for most of a therapy hour and only connect with an underlying feeling of rage at the very end. She may then be afraid that she could destroy anything in her path and find herself unable to return to work for hours afterward. She may want to talk to the therapist about the intensity and vulnerability of her feelings and to have the therapist understand them. Yet, if the therapist attempts to understand in a way that doesn't catch her feelings in exactly the right words, she may feel intensely violated by her therapist and cut off contact' (Warner, 2001, p.182).

'Maybe, if there was a lack of empathy in childhood, I don't know. His mother was there for him and perhaps she supplied the empathy, at least enough for him to not develop the potential to enter into fragile process. Hmm. I'm just thinking about how Gary is. It's difficult. He doesn't have the tone of that kind of fragility in the sessions. Yes, he's volatile but I'm not really seeing it, not to that degree. And, of course, the alcohol I am sure complicates it as well. It can increase volatility but it can depress the central nervous system as well, flattening functioning, if you like. But for Gary, though, it seems clear that alcohol increases his volatility, or at least his capacity to live out of an aggressive part of himself.'

'And that's an interesting way of looking at it, as if part of himself carries the aggression.'

'I suppose I sense that maybe as well as symbolising a need to never be like his father, he has somehow also established within his self-concept a need to be aggressive ...' Rick paused. 'Hmm, a thought, he talked last time about having to keep out of his father's way. I wonder if he has symbolised in some way the notion of having to be aggressive in order not to be threatened, intimidated, feel weak, a reaction to his father's behaviour towards him and his mother?'

Jean listened. 'Mhmm.'

Rick shook his head. 'I keep coming back to feeling that Gary's in for a rough phase if he has to confront an idea that he has become like his father. But he is defended against this. He sees his violence and aggression as having a purpose, whereas his father's seemed, well, unreasoned.' He went quiet, thinking now about person-centred theory and what happens when a self-concept comes under threat. 'It may be me getting defensive now, but my thoughts have gone to what Rogers said about what happens when the self-concept is threatened. Anxiety, but potentially more devastating effects.'

'In extreme cases, psychotic breakdown, you mean, as the self-concept is fractured.'

Rick nodded, aware that he had tightened his lips. He guessed it would be devastating for Gary to see himself as having some traits similar to his father, if that happened, but he was a unique individual, having his own distinctive reasons for his way of being. Yes, maybe the potential was there for Gary's alcohol use to become more established and perhaps, in time, develop into more of a full-blown dependency. Now, it seemed, it was dependent in relation to his need to feel and express aggression. And, of course, it was also in part an aspect of the social/drinking culture with which Gary identified himself. It wasn't all down to his father's influence. That would be far too simplistic. He expressed his thoughts to Jean.

'Yes, you are right. We must not lose sight of the complexity and the many factors and, as you say, Gary's own distinct uniqueness as a person. I was struck by what you said about whether you were thinking about theory as a defence of your own.'

Rick smiled. 'As a way of maybe not acknowledging the potential impact on Gary. But I cannot interfere in his process. My role is to be there for him, with him, listen to him, accept him, try and maintain an atmosphere of transparency, and trust, yes, that's the key, trust the process. Such a cliché and yet it isn't, it really isn't, it goes to the very heart of the therapy that we offer as person-centred practitioners, you know?'

Jean nodded. 'Trusting the process, at the heart of what we do.'

'It's a kind of therapeutic attitude, isn't it? I mean, it's not clearly defined as a necessary and sufficient condition for constructive personality change, but it is sort of implied. I couldn't function as a person-centred practitioner if I distrusted the process, I mean the process that is occuring in the client … well, and the therapeutic relational process as well, but it feels more about trusting, what, the actualising tendency isn't it, how it will shape – is that the right word –

what happens for, to, within Gary. It's hard to be sure of the right words.' He snorted as another thought came to mind. Jean noted this and raised her eyebrows, moving her head slightly, inviting Rick to express himself.

'And he's going to get anxious, and, yeah, I guess, so am I. Anxious for him. That's, hmm, is that OK? Should I be anxious if I trust the process?'

'That's the question it leaves you with, should you be anxious if you trust the process?'

'I suppose it's a different kind of anxiety. Maybe anxious isn't the right word, maybe concerned, linked to knowing he may be about to pass through something uncomfortable … hmm.' He paused, another thought. 'But maybe not as uncomfortable as what he has experienced in the past and, well, maybe something necessary for him to perhaps have an easier future, perhaps?'

'Mhmm. A sort of necessary experience for him?'

'And I'm a sort of catalyst in a way. Not intentionally trying to make anything happen, and maybe it would have happened anyway, but the therapeutic experience – the relational experience – is probably encouraging shifts within Gary, opening his awareness to possibilities. Tough experience, therapy, isn't it? You hear people talk about therapy being a soft option. That gets my goat. But even worse are those who say person-centred is somehow even more of a soft option because we're all being nice to our clients. What crap!'

Jean was struck by the sudden intensity in what Rick was saying, and the shift of focus. 'Sounds like that really gets to you, huh?'

Rick shook his head. 'Soft option my eye. Offering a relational experience, therapeutic conditions, that encourage clients to come face to face with their own incongruence, a soft option?' He shook his head. 'Bloody hard work, for client and person-centred therapist. Sometimes there's this idea that we just sit and listen. JUST SIT AND LISTEN! Maybe if a few more people had sat and listened we wouldn't have so many people needing to pay for someone to listen to them.' Rick could feel his own intensity. It wasn't that he didn't enjoy his work, he did, he really did, but he also wished sometimes that there was greater recognition of the discipline of the person-centred approach to counselling, psychotherapy, that it was a genuine psychological approach, rigorously researched, Rogers and many of his colleagues having been very much involved in applying scientific methodology to researching and understanding what they were offering and what was effective. He sat back in the chair. 'Tell Gary this is a soft option!'

'Mhmm, for him, for you …'

'I just wish that there was a greater recognition of what we are doing. We know that the relationship is crucial, that empathy is a key feature of effective

therapy, whatever the approach. I just know in myself that relational therapy – I sometimes call it that – is what so many young people could benefit
from. Spending time with people who are open and honest with them, who
listen to them, take them seriously, accept them for who they are, what they
are, how they are. We live in a society that feels at times so dehumanising.
So much of the entertainment is loud and in your face, intense. Kids put in
front of the TV, watching videos, playing computer games, being entertained
electronically. Where's the human contact? No wonder kids can't contain
feelings, and get out of order. I reckon there's something really powerful in
what Margaret Warner says about fragile process and its origin in a kind of
empathy deprivation. I think it's more widespread than we think. I suspect
it's behind a lot of so-called psychiatric or psychological syndromes, maybe
even attention deficit disorder, I don't know. Lack of empathy and junk food.
Oh well, time to get off my soapbox. I'm a bit like Gary, at the end of the last
session he thanked me for listening and how he'd needed to get a few things
off his chest.'
'You too. And I think you're making some really valid points. It's like – and I
know we're getting away from supervision perhaps – but it's like society is in
an incongruent state, denying to awareness that there are facets of society that
are actually causing the problems we complain about. We have a kind of
collective self-concept of being a healthy society – Western society is good,
consumer societies are healthy – but there are experiences pressing in on our
awareness, threatening our self-concept. In fact we are a very unhealthy
society, physically, emotionally, mentally, and I would say spiritually. Is there
a collective self-concept in society and what happens when that is threatened?'
'Anxiety, stress, confusion, probably greater volatility, desperation and clinging
to habits that you don't want to accept as being unhealthy, so maybe addic-
tions become more intense and more things become focuses of addiction. Shit,
that sounds too close, doesn't it?' Rick was shaking his head. 'And there are
young people developing in this world, trying to make sense of themselves,
trying to find a place in a social order riddled with incongruence. You know,
at a societal level, it's no wonder there is so much drug and alcohol use. And
binge drinking, young people doing what they need to do to get an experience.
In a way it's like taking control although we know it means losing control. But
with alcohol you know what you'll get. It's reliable. Drink a lot, you have a few
laughs, you get pissed. Yeah, you may do things you later regret, but somehow
that's not a barrier. The urge is too strong. The fix too intense.' Rick felt himself
go quiet, he felt emotional. 'I want to listen. I want to make a difference. I want
to provide some kind of therapeutic oasis in the midst of this crazy world.'
Jean nodded. 'Mhmm, you care, you want to make a difference, give people a
place on the oasis.'
'Yeah. Hadn't expected to get to this, but yeah. I can't change Gary, and, well,
no, I can't. And I don't want to try and change him in any particular way.
He will change if he is ready in whatever way is right for him. But I am clear
that I do want to offer him the therapeutic conditions so that, should the
time be right, he can make the choices he needs to make and hopefully

from a place of experiencing a more realistic – perhaps I should say congruent – sense of self.'

'And that's it, isn't it? You put that really clearly. We offer a relational/therapeutic experience and trust what emerges.'

Rick nodded. He felt good to have raged a bit and had his rant. Releasing it had brought him back to what really mattered, what was present for him, what motivated him, and what would ensure that he did the best he could to be a person-centred therapist in relationship with his clients. He was also aware of another theme now present in his thinking, and he voiced this as he wanted to acknowledge and explore Gary's actual alcohol use.

'Another theme I do want to touch on here is in relation to Gary's alcohol use.'

'Mhmm, what about it?'

'Well, as you know, as a person-centred therapist I am seeking to offer the therapeutic conditions and trust him to bring to the session what is pressing for him, or whatever he wants to explore. We haven't explored his drinking pattern that much or the amount that he drinks, and I want to acknowledge that. I guess because, well, in the world of alcohol counselling there is so much emphasis on, for instance, motivational approaches, and yet by working with clients the way that I do I believe that their motivation *is* something that is worked with, but not directly as a kind of specified issue. I want my clients, if they are going to be motivated to change, to be so because *they* see the need, or experience a dissatisfaction with how things are and want change, not because someone else is telling them to change, or encouraging them to change perhaps in a way that may take them beyond what they are genuinely ready for and able to own. Does that make sense?'

'Mhmm, it does, the idea that by directly motivating a person to change a drinking pattern, for instance, may not be matched by, or perhaps we should say congruent with, their own inner experiencing.'

'Their own relationship with, well, yes, as in this case, alcohol. I always come back to sustainable change and my sense that unless the person changes constructively – that's the way person-centred theory describes it – then behaviour and indeed cognitive change is less likely to be sustainable. The way we behave, the way we see things are a product of who we are, how we experience ourselves, the experiences that we allow into our awareness and those that we deny to awareness – this is the primary focus; behaviour and cognition flow from this, and, of course, they also provide feedback as well to reinforce our self-concept. It's, yes, I suppose what I am wanting to say is that perhaps motivational work, in attempting to change cognition and behaviour that is out of step with what the client is ready for, that is not in tune with the working of their own actualising tendency, could enforce a disruption of the client's self-concept and, well, hmm, maybe this is extreme, but if we think about what Rogers said about this, about the disorganisation that can develop as a result of incongruence entering awareness, then, well, I just wonder if in some cases it could lead to psychotic breakdown or, at least, a degree of disorganisation that someone may not then have the therapeutic knowledge and understanding to enable the client to work through.'

Rogers wrote of the process of psychological breakdown and disorganisation. He expressed four stages to this process, the first two stages of which 'may be illustrated by anxiety-producing experiences in therapy, or by acute psychotic breakdowns'.

1 'If the individual has a large or significant degree of *incongruence between self and experience*, and if a significant experience demonstrating this *incongruence* occurs suddenly, or with a high degree of obviousness, then the organism's process of *defense* is unable to operate successfully.

2 As a result *anxiety is experienced*, as the *incongruence* is subceived. The degree of anxiety is dependent upon the extent of the *self-structure* which is *threatened*'(Rogers, 1959, pp. 228–9).

As a result of this process, Rogers then went on to describe the effects this has on the individual's self-structure and subsequent behaviour. He writes:

3 'The process of defense being unsuccessful, the *experience* is *accurately symbolised* in *awareness*, and the gestalt of the *self-structure* is broken by this *experience* of the *incongruence* in *awareness*. A state of disorganisation results.

4 In such a state of disorganisation the organism behaves at times in ways which are openly consistent with experiences which have hitherto been distorted or denied to awareness. At other times the self may temporarily regain regnancy, and the organism may behave in ways consistent with it. Thus in such a state of disorganisation, the tension between the concept of self (with its included distorted perceptions) and the experiences which are not accurately symbolised or included in the concept of self, is expressed in a confused regnancy, first one and then the other supplying the "feedback" by which the organism regulates behaviour' (Rogers, 1959, pp. 229).

'Interesting thought. I can see where you are coming from. Is this something you think Gary is at risk from, then, if, say, he had seen someone that had sought to let's say make him see that his drinking and behaviour is close to that of his father?' Jean could appreciate what Rick was saying. She felt there wasn't enough understanding of the impact of changes that someone might be subject to, but which they were genuinely not ready or able to symbolise into their awareness in such a way that they could genuinely identify with that need for change.

'I don't know, but I can see the risk and that what would happen is Gary may not be able to sustain maintaining the incongruence in his awareness and would either have to, say, drink more to try to blank it out, break contact with therapy because it was simply too threatening to his sense of self, or, yes, if he could be offered a therapeutic relationship to support him in his process, then maybe he would be able to symbolise accurately his new perception into his awareness and adjust his self-concept, or adjust his behaviour so that he did not need to do this, of course.' Rick paused, he hadn't planned to say so much, indeed he had originally simply wanted to make some comment about how they weren't talking much about what Gary was actually drinking. But it had felt good to talk the way that he had, it had helped him to connect more with his own thoughts, and clarify the risk that could come with a client being externally motivated beyond what they were ready for.

'Yes, it becomes a choice, and for me it is something about whether the client can identify with the need for that change, or with the different sense of self that changes in the way they think or behave might encourage. And, yes, as Rogers said, when incongruence breaks into awareness, there will be times when different perspectives are held at the same time, the client oscillating between them.'

'In Gary's case it could become a sense that he is like his father, which would trigger a set of thoughts, feelings and behaviours, while at other times this would be denied to awareness and another set of thoughts, feelings and behaviours would be present and, of course, there may well be overlaps as well.' Rick stopped, wanting to take a moment to consider where he was in all of this. How did it leave him feeling? What were the challenges to him, for him, in working with Gary?

'Mhmm, with him moving between them.'

Rick nodded, still with his own thoughts. 'And that's the challenge, isn't it, for me, to be able to honour – yes, that's a good word – honour both sets of feelings, thoughts. It's not a word we often use, we talk about unconditional positive regard, and maybe respect as well, but there is something about *honouring* what is present for the client. And I am also very aware of a sense of uncertainty, of not knowing how things will work out for Gary, or for that matter how it will be as far as the therapeutic relationship is concerned.' He lapsed momentarily into silence. 'The challenge is to not be directive, not allow my hopes for Gary to affect my responses. Directiveness isn't so much about what we do or say as it is about attitude and intention, wouldn't you say?'

Jean nodded. 'Motivation. Why we say what we say. Are we trying to make something happen, or are we maintaining our focus on the client's inner world that they are communicating to us and being open to what occurs, whatever it may be?'

'It's not easy, working with a person with their life ahead of them, seeing them in effect trapping themselves in a set of behaviours, even though they have meaning for that person. I kind of think it is harder to remain non-directive in these circumstances. It's so tempting, and I'm sure I don't manage 100% non-directivity. I'm sure there are times when what I say or the way I say it carries a direction. And, yes, maybe the intent isn't there, but maybe sometimes it is as well. And that's what I need to be sensitive to and ensure that I keep my focus on my client, on Gary, and allow the actualising tendency – the power within his own self – to direct him. And that's what I have to come back to.'

'The actualising tendency?'

Rick nodded. 'That is at the heart of the approach, that core belief, maybe more than a belief, a knowing, that there is an actualising tendency at work and that it can be trusted. I have to give Gary the therapeutic relational experience that will, well, contribute to the possibility of constructive personality change.' He paused again. 'It's good to talk like this, have time to connect with the essence of what we do, what I do. I form therapeutic relationship, that's my job, if you like, what I suppose I'm an expert in, what I am motivated to do, and it is satisfying, there's no doubt about that, to be part of a therapeutic relationship. Everything sharpens down into the relationship. It can be such an intense experience. Maybe almost addictive! You sort of feel you're working alongside or with some greater process. It's personal and yet there's something universal about it as well. The actualising tendency is in everyone – is "in" the right word? And it's everywhere if we take Rogers' idea of a formative tendency at work in everything from crystals to stars, throughout nature. I feel sort of restored talking like this. Ready to go back into the world, as it were, with a sort of restored sense of what I am about. That feels good.'

'Feels good to me, too.' Jean smiled back. 'That's a part of supervision and I'm glad that you experience it. And I am sure it contributes to your effectiveness as a therapist as well, of course.'

The supervision session moved on as Rick realised he needed to mention another client who had suddenly stopped attending. Somehow the broken contact with that client suddenly felt sharper after the conversation he had been having and the experience that had become present for him. It was like a sharp disconnection against a backdrop of connectedness, and he wanted to explore it further.

Points for discussion

- Assess the value of this supervision session. What key areas were addressed?
- How were the attitudes and values of the person-centred approach offered by the supervisor?
- What else might have been brought to this supervision session?
- How do you react to the comments about society? What do you feel about the notion of a kind of 'collective self-concept' and the idea that incongruence is impacting on awareness?
- What are your thoughts in response to the exploration about change towards the end of this session? How do you assess the impact and implications of change in behaviour and cognition beyond what the client can accurately symbolise and sustain in awareness?
- What do you see as the effect that this supervision session has had on Rick and what key points might he take away from it?

CHAPTER 6

Counselling session 6: alcohol use has increased and an emotional release

Wednesday 21 May

'I want to drink ... and I don't want to drink.' Gary paused, he was confused. 'Does that make sense?'

'You want to drink, you feel that urge clearly, but you also feel an urge not to drink as well. Two very different experiences.' Rick felt it did make sense and he hoped his empathic response conveyed the sense that he felt from what Gary had been saying.

'I feel really unsettled, *really* unsettled. Keep thinking about the past, that makes me want to drink. And then ...' He shook his head, 'then I really feel bad, I don't know, like I can't ...' He shook his head again, not knowing what to say.

'You feel bad, like you can't ...?'

'Like I can't sort of, I don't know, I don't like myself. I don't like that I keep wanting a drink. It's not a laugh any more. I mean, it sort of is, but it isn't, not really. Mal and Luke have both said I need to ease back, that I'm getting a pain, going moody, causing trouble. That's what they said. Bevvied up again over the weekend, you know, got stuck in a couple of times. I just lose it. And it's getting worse. It feels like it's getting worse. I feel worse, feel fucking awful. Just want to drink. Ended up drinking through Sunday, didn't go into work Monday, too pissed. Didn't care. Didn't want to fucking know. That's how I feel. Just feel fucked up. Don't know what to do, 'cept have another drink.' He shrugged. 'It's no good, is it? I'll become like my old man.'

'That's what it feels like, Gary, that you'll become like your old man?'

Gary was staring down. He hadn't meant to say it, but it was something he'd been thinking about and he didn't like what he was thinking. He knew he was different, and yet, it troubled him, and had done more and more that past week. He'd left the last session feeling OK, thoughtful, yeah, but OK. Felt he'd said what he wanted to say, but he'd felt different as well. Like he was seeing things differently, seeing himself differently. Not something he'd really thought about at

97

the time, but now, and as the week had gone on, he could see the alcohol was a problem, but he still wanted a drink. That was the thing, more than anything else, that was leaving him wondering, and feeling uncomfortable.

Gary continued looking down, saying nothing. He bit his lip. He felt stiff. Couldn't feel comfortable in the chair. Moved himself around a bit; it didn't help. He wished he could get his old man out of his head. Only the drink seemed to help, he forgot things then, got into the business of drinking and having a few laughs, except he didn't feel much like laughing. He just felt angry, pissed off, sorry for himself, really, more that than anything else. Just breathing seemed to take an effort. And he felt tired. He'd thought about some pills to give himself a boost, but that wasn't what he needed. He knew that. Just screw him up even more. No, he needed to get a grip on himself, but he didn't know how.

Thud, smack, shouting, his mother screaming. He closed his eyes. The sounds wouldn't go away. His jaw tightened. He'd kill the bastard if he got hold of him now, he was bloody sure he would. It always felt good hitting out, giving someone a kicking.

He took a deep breath. 'I feel like it's him I'm fighting, you know?'

'Like you're fighting your old man?'

Gary nodded. 'Like I'm trying to, I don't know, kick him out of my head. It's him I want to lay into, he's the one. I'm just so fed up with it all. I can't go on like this.'

The thought flashed through Rick's mind – is he suicidal? Young male heavy drinkers have a high incidence of suicide. But that may not have been what Gary was thinking. Rick didn't know. He stayed with what Gary had said and the way he had said it.

'Feels like you can't go on the way you are at the moment.'

'I need a life, I need to move on, I need to ...' He shook his head, not knowing exactly what he needed, but he knew things had to be different. 'Coming here, yeah, I talk about things, things I don't talk to anyone else about, things that, well, I don't feel too good about, you know? I've told you stuff that I haven't said to anyone else. It's different here. It's good, but ...' he was shaking his head again. 'But I feel worse, you know? I don't understand.'

'Yeah, coming here, talking to me like you do, and you end up feeling worse, yeah. And that's what you don't understand.'

'I'm drinking more, fighting more, feeling more fucked up. I want it to be different.'

'Mhmm, you want it to be different. You don't want to drink more, fight more or feel more fucked up. You've had enough of it.' Rick felt he had empathised, though perhaps he had upped the emphasis in his response. But he didn't feel he was saying anything that was out of touch with what Gary had been saying.

'Yeah. Not that I want to go back to how it was, I mean, it was still a problem, I guess. I don't know, I just want to be different. Is that too much to ask?'

'Is it too much to ask to be different?'

'Feels like it. But I have to, I know it.' He lifted his hands to his face and rubbed. He felt hot. He hadn't really got over the weekend's drinking. He belched. 'Sorry.'

'Feels like you have to change.'

Gary sat with his discomfort, wishing he could have a drink, and wishing he didn't want to have a drink at the same time. 'You were right, I have got a problem. I didn't want to hear it. I still don't, but I can't go on drinking and getting into fights. I know I can handle it, but I have to do it, don't I? I've got to prove it to myself.' He also thought about his mum. She'd been telling him that he needed to do something about his drinking. He didn't like to upset her, but he knew that he did. She was the one person who cared, she'd had it rough but she was OK now, had a good set of friends and that was, yeah, good to see. 'I'm not like him. I just, well, yeah, drink too much sometimes and, yeah . . .' He shrugged.

'That's all it is, just drink too much sometimes . . . ?'

'I'm not an alcy, and I'll never be an alcy.'

'Mhmm, no, that's something you're not and you don't ever want to be.'

'I like feeling pissed, though, you know? Doesn't everyone?'

'That's how it seems, you like getting pissed and it seems that everyone does as well.'

'Well, yeah, most people, you know?'

'Maybe, maybe not, but you see it as most people.'

'Why do I fucking do it?' Gary slammed his fist down on the arm of the chair. The explosive reaction took Rick by surprise. He could see the anger and the frustration on Gary's face. 'I don't want to be like this. I need to get a fucking grip. For fuck's sake, why can't I get him out of my fucking head?'

'Your father?'

Gary started to nod, but he could feel emotion surging into his body, his throat dry and tight, he swallowed; his eyes filling with water, he blinked. He took a deep breath, it was faltering. He swallowed again. It was a struggle. His eyes were stinging, his throat felt as though it had a large lump in it and he couldn't shift it. He sniffed and rubbed his face. He felt hot and very uncomfortable. He felt anxious, small – that was weird, but yeah, he felt small. Like he was sort of . . . , he couldn't make sense of it, and he didn't want to try. It was how he was, feeling small. He swallowed again, he found it hard to breathe. He was getting hotter, his hands, lower arms felt a strange tingly numbness. 'Why? Why?' The word kept coming out of his mouth. He had no answer. He didn't understand. And he was now left feeling like shit, screwed up, fucked up. He knew a few drinks would sort it, and it wouldn't. Just leave him wanting more. And he'd do something stupid anyway. He felt his jaw tightening, his teeth jammed together. His fists were tight as he sat in the chair. He was looking down at them. He could feel a kind of jerkiness in his body. He tightened and relaxed his fists, again and again. He could feel his nails digging into his palms. Each time it felt like he was tightening them more, tightening his arms. It was like he was trying to hold himself together. All he could think about was how he hated his old man, how he'd been, what he'd done to him and to his mum. He could feel his body trembling, shaking, as he tightened up. He held the tightness, the shaking grew. He could feel it in his upper arms, his shoulders, in his chest. He breathed through his nose, he could hear the breath coming in and out. His head was bowed. He leaned forward bringing his fists up to his face, his thumbs against his lips, now his breathing came in short sharp breaths. He was quite oblivious of the room around him, and of the fact that that was how he sat as a child, in his room, when he heard the fights, the thuds, his mother's screams, her crying, his father's angry voice, shouting, always shouting.

Rick looked on. Gary's head was bowed so far down, he continued to shake. Rick didn't want to interrupt what was happening. Clearly Gary was connecting with strong feelings, and it was clearly in his body. The physicality of what was happening for Gary was so present in the room. Rick wanted to let Gary know that he was there, that he, Gary, was not alone with his experiencing, but equally he didn't want to disrupt the process and risk taking Gary's focus away from what was happening. He spoke gently. He didn't know exactly what Gary was experiencing, but he could imagine that it had to be linked to things that Gary had experienced. Either that or it was a reaction to his dilemma in the present. He decided to respond in a way that could encompass both. 'A horrible, horrible experience.'

Gary heard Rick's voice but it seemed very distant, like it was outside his reality. It was horrible, yes, it was, but he wasn't in a place in himself to think about it. He was too full of what he was feeling. No space to think about it. He was what he was feeling, it filled him. So many feelings, scared, so scared. So small, and so scared. He had begun to rock, to and fro in the chair, only slightly, hardly aware himself that he was doing it.

Rick noticed the movement. It was not uncommon for children to rock when they were frightened, traumatised by something. He sought to empathise with what he felt Gary might be experiencing, wanting to keep in contact with him. His thought was that perhaps, in the past, Gary would have been very much alone. Now, well, now he could be aware that someone was there with him, for him. 'Frightening, so frightening.' He immediately wondered if that was the right word. Maybe terrifying. Maybe. But what age might Gary be re-experiencing his feelings from? What words would he have related to at that age? He didn't know. No point in speculating. He knew his intention was to reach out to him. He felt sadness in his heart, and a compassion for this young man who had suddenly, or so it seemed, become the terror that he had known in the past.

Gary felt the tension in his body ease, his breathing became easier as well and he lifted up his head. His eyes were closed. He leaned back in the chair, lifting his hands on to the top of his head. Rick noticed him screw his eyes up tighter as he did so. He let out a long breath through his nose and breathed in through his mouth, letting it out, blowing it out through his mouth. He opened his eyes, looking up towards the ceiling. Another deep breath and again blowing out the air through his mouth. He felt calmer, as if something had been released, let go of. His arms ached, his chest felt sore. He brought his hands down and rubbed his chest. He winced. It was painful to rub, it felt like his rib cage was stiff with pain. 'Oh Jeez.' He blinked, taking another deep breath. He could feel his ribs moving as he did so. He flexed his shoulders back a little to try to release the stiffness. 'Oh shit. What the hell happened there? Fuck, I feel stiff.'

He stretched again. 'Bloody hell.' Another deep breath. He rubbed his eyes and shook his head. 'Crazy as it sounds, I sort of feel better for that. But I feel bloody knackered.' His eyes felt heavy, like he'd used up all the energy that he needed to keep his eyes open. His head felt strangely empty. Weird thing to think, but that was how it was.

Rick sat and sought to empathise with what Gary was saying and experiencing. 'Knackering, huh, all that emotion?'

Gary burped and felt a sudden pain in his chest as he did so. 'I feel like all my muscles are, Jeez, so fucking tight.' He touched his ribs again. 'Fuck!' Bloody hell, they're sore, he thought to himself. He was shaking his head again. Felt like the only bit of his upper body he could move that didn't feel sore. He was taking another deep breath, and then he spoke again. 'What the hell was that? I just, I don't know, I just felt . . . , I can't explain. Just so tight, and so afraid. Frightening, yeah, and horrible, but more than that. Terror, just . . .' He couldn't find the words. He could feel himself frowning and his eyes filling with water. 'I was so afraid, so, so . . . , I don't know, just stuck, I couldn't . . .' He paused and then tried to speak, but didn't know what to say. He couldn't find the words to describe it. He didn't know how to describe it, it felt too big, too . . . He shrugged and blew out another deep breath.

'Hard to describe, so afraid, so stuck . . .' Rick kept his response simple and to the words that Gary had used. It was a sensitive time. He didn't want to lead Gary into a vocabulary that was not his own, or lead him into finding words that might not really be those that Gary wanted to use. He wanted to keep his empathy clear and focused on what Gary was saying.

Where clients are struggling to find the right words to describe what they are feeling, it is vital that the counsellor stays with what the client is saying. If more words are introduced, it can direct the client towards thinking about their experience when in fact their process may be simply requiring them to be with, or to be, what they are feeling. The visceral focus is maintained, and a lurch into cognitive processing is avoided. The inner world and the inner experience of the client that is present and experienced is respected, and warm acceptance is conveyed.

Gary was shaking his head again, and blinking. 'Trapped. No way out. That's how it was. Trapped, listening, hating it, wanting it to stop. Just wanting it to stop.'

Rick nodded, feeling a stinging in his own eyes and a heaviness in his own heart. He felt himself taking a deep breath himself, suddenly aware of how tense he had become in his body as he had sat listening and attending to his client. 'Yeah, just wanting it to stop.'

There was something about the way Rick spoke that struck a chord with Gary. It had sounded almost like a kind of sigh, and that was how it felt for him. Just-wanting-it-to-stop, wanting it to all just go away, not happen. That's how it had been, and how it had felt just now. So real, so close, like it was happening, really happening, and now.

'It didn't though. Not every night, but most nights, particularly Fridays and Saturdays. Sometimes friends would ask me to sleep over. I wanted to, but I was afraid to. Afraid what would happen when I wasn't there. But I couldn't do anything.' Gary was sitting back in the chair, his forearms at an angle on the arm rests. His lips pursed once more. His arms felt heavy, he felt heavy in the chair. Yeah, it was like all the energy had gone out of his body.

'You talked about feeling trapped.'

'Trapped at home, trapped having to be home.' He shook his head and took a deep breath, feeling his chest expand as he did so, and noting that the soreness had eased a little. His mouth was dry. 'Have you any water?'

'Yeah, sure, I'll get some.' Rick went out to the water dispenser and filled up a cup. He brought one back for himself as well. He handed one cup to Gary and took a sip from the other. It felt cool in his mouth and throat.

'Was that, well, I mean, was that normal, what just happened to me?'

'It can happen like that. It's different for everyone, of course, but it can happen.'

'Felt like it was in me, more than in me, it *was me*.'

'Like you were reliving it for real?'

'Yeah, yeah, that's exactly it.' Gary frowned. 'How can that be? I mean, do you carry that sort of stuff around with you? Is that it? Have I had that inside me all the time? Is it still there? Has it gone, can I get rid of it?'

Rick wasn't sure what to say. He didn't really have an answer. How did you explain it? Did it go, or was it always there? 'I don't know, Gary, I don't know. People experience it differently. How do you feel now?'

'Calmer, tired, not sure what to make of it all. Feel like I need to go somewhere really quiet. And I don't feel like a drink!'

'You sound surprised?'

Gary nodded. 'Yeah, well, yeah, you'd think I would, you know? But it's not the answer, is it? I mean, if that's what I've had locked up inside me, Jesus.' A thought struck him and he was voicing it before he had a chance to really think about it. 'No wonder I explode!'

Rick felt himself smile. He nodded. 'Yeah, no wonder you explode.'

'That's it, isn't it? Me, needing to explode and trying not to, but having to. That's what I do, don't I? That's what I've been doing for a while now. Getting angry, pissed off, frustrated, blowing up.' He was shaking his head again, slowly, trying to really grasp what he was saying. He looked at Rick. 'That is it, isn't it? You knew it, didn't you? But you could have told me. I wouldn't have believed you, understood it.' He looked away and snorted, shaking his head again.

'Probably not. We can only grasp what we can, when we can. It's always more powerful when we see things for ourselves, when we make sense of things in our way.'

Gary nodded, and looked back at Rick, looking deeply into his eyes. 'It's why I drink, isn't it?'

Rick nodded. It felt the most congruent response. He didn't say anything, Gary had said it himself. Best to leave him with the sound of his own words.

'What now?'

'What do you want now?'

'Sort myself out. Get myself back on track. Get a grip on things. And, yeah, I wanna talk to my mum.'

'Sounds good to me. Trust yourself, trust yourself to know what you need to do.'

Gary nodded. Yeah, that sounded good. He even felt that maybe he could. 'Yeah.' He lapsed into momentary silence. 'Won't be easy, though.'

'No.'

'It's been tough getting here, still got to work at it, yeah?'

'Yeah.'

'Hmm.' Gary took a deep breath. Rick wasn't saying much, but then, well, he didn't need to. It was kind of clear. It wasn't going to be easy and it had been tough. He had to get his drinking under control. It somehow seemed so much clearer to him all of a sudden. He glanced over at the clock. The session was due to end.

Rick noticed the glance. 'You feeling OK to end this session?'

'Yeah.' He paused. 'Still trying to make sense of it.'

'Mhmm. Lot to make sense of. It's been intense. Just ease yourself quietly back into the day. You'll feel in quite a sensitive state for a while. Look after yourself, yeah?'

Gary nodded, taking a deep breath, 'Yeah. Yeah, I can see that. I almost don't want to go to work. Maybe I won't hurry, take my time. I can say I got stuck in traffic.'

'OK, so, next week?'

'Yeah. Yeah, thanks. Never thought it'd be like this, never imagined. But, yeah, it's good, guess it's what I needed, what I need. Got to make some changes, haven't I?'

'Only if you want to.'

'I do. Yeah.' Gary got up and headed out the door, still aware of feeling sort of disconnected somehow, well, not with himself, more with his surroundings. It all felt so intense. He walked slowly back along the corridor towards the exit, as Rick returned to the counselling room to reflect on the session and write his notes.

Points for discussion

- How has this session left you feeling?
- Was there anything that Rick did that seemed to facilitate what happened for Gary in that session?
- How would you summarise what has happened in this session from a person-centred theoretical viewpoint?
- Thinking back over the sessions that Gary has had with Rick, what seem to you to be the key moments, and why?
- What do you think will be Gary's main challenge now in the coming weeks? What processes will he have to deal with?
- What might you take from this session to supervision?

Write notes for this session.

Reflections

It's a few weeks later, the counselling process has continued with Gary attending regularly. He's relived more of his past experiences and has been working at changing his drinking. It hasn't been easy. Some success and a few slips along the way. Nothing unusual about that. His motivation has been very much still linked to not wanting to be like his father. As it became clearer to him that he was at risk of being like him, that need to be different became stronger, more present. From a person-centred perspective one might think of it as having become a focus for the actualising tendency. His need to not be like his father became the drive towards a more satisfying sense of himself. He began to stop denying the possibility that his behaviour had similarities.

Rick didn't try to make him become different, but difference emerged as a result of the therapeutic encounters that they were having. Gradually Gary began to change his lifestyle, though he didn't stop drinking. He didn't want that. He could see that he drank to get angry to express himself, release the pent-up emotion within him. And that some of it was a kind of learned behaviour. He became more aware of hating how he had become. He found it hard to accept himself, to feel genuine positive self-regard. He used to have it, or what he thought was it. Though in fact really he was behaving in ways so that he felt he was respected by others, and it was that which made him feel good.

What he was having to learn was to not rely on others for his self-esteem, but to be able to feel good about himself, within himself. That wasn't easy.

Gary considers his counselling experience

'None of this was what I expected. I really wasn't too sure of Rick to start with. Certainly didn't want to be there. It's taken a while for me to realise that, yeah, I do have a problem, and to begin to see why. Makes me angry, probably always will. Maybe it'll change. At the moment I'm not sure that I want to stop being angry, particularly at my old man, for what he was, what he did to mum, and to me.

I mean, yeah, I suppose you could say he had his reasons, but he was out of order. You can't justify it, you know? And I don't want to get like that, and, well, yeah, I can see that while I'm not like him, I've got out of order too. I've still got some way to go to understanding it all, but I want to now. Yeah, it troubles me that maybe there are parts of me that are like him. I don't want that.

So much drinking goes on, you know, Friday night, Saturday night, every night for those that can afford it. Crazy, but that's how it is. Maybe not for everyone, I can see that more clearly now, you can make different choices, but it's not easy. Everywhere you go there's alcohol. You just drink, don't think about it as a problem. It's what you do, what your mates do, have a few laughs, it's what life's about. At least, that's how it seemed, now I'm not so sure. Now I'm not sure if that's what I really want. What'll I have to show for it? Just get more fucked up.

But life's about having a good time. That's what it is. Enjoy yourself, now. Stuff tomorrow, worry about that then. World's a mess anyway, who knows what tomorrow'll be like? No, fuck tomorrow, enjoy today. Except . . . I don't know. Now I'm not so sure. Drinking, fighting, yeah, felt good, felt right, know what I mean? Never knew any different. Brought up on it I suppose. Fighting, you had to, get respect, yeah, get a reputation. Made me feel good, course it did. Doesn't any more, not the same. I'm beginning to feel different. Can't really explain it.

It's like it's so in your head. What you do. You stand your ground, that's how it is. Keep feeling good, do what it takes, fuck everyone else, except your mates, of course. At least, that's how it's been for me. Probably not like that for everyone. Some people had it better than me, didn't learn the kind of stuff I had to learn to get by. Does that make 'em any better than me? You don't have to have a crap childhood to want to get pissed. It's how it was for me. But not everyone's like that.

It's hard to think it can be different. It's so in your head. Counselling's helped me to get stuff out of my head, and not just my head. Shit, it's been tough. Still is. But I sort of know now that I've got to carry on. I can't go back, though it's tempting at times. I mean, yeah, makes you wonder. It's like sort of waking up, but you kind of drift back as well. Weird really. Must be even harder for people who don't sort of try and change sooner. I mean, now, thinking about it, if I hadn't come to counselling, just carried on the way I was, I mean, then what? Probably be banged up in jail by now. Or worse. But you don't think like that at the time. It's just a laugh. You don't care. You really don't care. That's what people don't understand. You care what other people think about you – your mates that is, but anyone else? Fuck 'em. At least, that's how it was.

Kids are out there, eight, nine, ten, with this attitude. I guess I was like that, but I don't think I was bad. Not then. What'll they be like in ten years' time? They'll be worse than me. They're lippy, don't give a shit. We blame them. It'd be like blaming me, but I didn't know any different. Did what I had to do to survive, feel good, get respect. Yeah, did what I had to do, but it's worse, in just a few years, kids with knives, even guns. World gone fucking mad. There is something seriously wrong out there.

Makes me wonder. What would have made it different for me? Feel loved, I guess. Parents being there for me. Sounds kind of pissy to say it like that, but that's how I think it needed to be. Yeah, mum tried, course she did, and she was there, but she had problems of her own to sort out. Found it hard to be there for me. And the old man, well, he just fucked us both up. Chaos, fear, never knowing what was going to happen next, so you took control, control over what you could control, yourself, your own life, how other kids saw you.

Yeah, the more I think about it, yeah, I needed some kind of stability, people giving me time. Too many hours in front of the TV, maybe, I don't know. Living in a crap flat, always hassle around. Nothing to do. No money. Tension, always tension in the air. It becomes part of you. I don't know. What do the experts say? What do they know? Let them have my life, see if they'd be any different from me.

Anyway, yeah, now I'm trying to change. Feel like I've turned a bit of a corner. But got to keep at it. Looking back I guess what really helped me was having someone to listen. Wasn't sure about it at first. Sometimes I felt like I wasn't sort of accepted somehow. Maybe that was my stuff, looking for reasons to not want to be there. But, yeah, Rick listens. Crazy isn't it, but that's it, he listens. Gives me time. Gives me respect, but it's different, not the sort of respect I'm used to. Don't really understand it, but now I've got used to it, yeah, it's good. Wish someone like him had been around earlier in my life. I'm sure things would have been different. That's it though, isn't it, having someone there for you, someone who, yeah, takes you seriously, and sits with you, helps you make sense of things. Like I say, mum tried, but she had her own demons to sort out.

So, yeah, not been easy, still isn't, still trying to get the crap out of my head. I know I want to. I'm realising things can be different, but it's not easy. Get bored easily. Find it hard to settle on things. Not sure what I'm going to do. But it's better than it was. Just have to see how it goes.'

Rick reflects on young people and binge drinking

'Some people have a tough start in life, and it is so easy to not see that when you are confronted with difficult behaviours in the present. There is so much emphasis on understanding why people end up struggling to cope with life and turn to drink and drugs, when the emphasis needs to be at least as much on what childhood experience they had, minimising the negative impact. I'm thinking of the factors that encourage resilience, which I know Richard Velleman has written about in order to enable the child or young person to have a less chaotic and disruptive experience, the role of the non-drinking parent, or a close relative, the family trying to present some degree of cohesion and consistency, for instance (Velleman, 1993, 1995; Orford and Velleman, 1995).

It feels to me as though Gary has made a breakthrough. Yes, his drinking got worse for a while, and that's not surprising, it was the one resource he had to cope with. He didn't have an internal resource to be able to face up to the feelings, the memories, the implications of his past on how he saw himself and his behaviour in the present. It feels as though we have connected more strongly now, much more of an alliance. Looking back, I know I struggled. I wasn't as good a counsellor as I would have liked to have been. At times my overwhelming sense of him as a young man with a problem, and why couldn't he see it, got the better of me. I don't like to see people, particularly young people, putting their health, their lives, their wellbeing at risk. That's me, and while it motivates me it can also get in the way of my empathy, and I have to keep working on that.

Yes, Gary's making progress. He's acknowledging his feelings and how the past has affected him, and he is making fresh choices in the present. OK, he's still drinking, but then his alcohol use is somewhat issue based, and while he may have begun to get close to chemical dependence (needing to drink alcohol to stave off withdrawal reactions), his main problem was psychological dependence (drinking to deal with, avoid or as an expression of psychological experience).

Of course, young people drink for many reasons, and it isn't always driven by early life experience. For many young people it is simply a habit that gets out of control, or the identifying with a particular culture which, over time, leads to alcohol becoming a dominant feature in a young person's life. So many people do drink these days to "get off their faces" and I do wonder what is it that drives this need. Is it clever advertising? Is it boredom and the need to release pent-up energy? Is it a need to alter mood? Is it just doing what everyone else seems to be doing because it's cool?

What has to be remembered is that each young person drinks for their own reason. It has its own meaning to them, its own part in their complex lifestyle. For Gary, alcohol was linked to his past experience, his emotional state, but also to his social experiencing and his need to see himself as someone who was strong, who dealt with things. It fed into a self-concept that had been shaped by early life experiences.

These factors seem to get forgotten when we read about "yob culture" and "binge drinking". Only the behaviour is made visible. I don't want to excuse alcohol-fuelled yobbish behaviour, but let's ask ourselves what is actually happening for these young people, what has shaped them to be the way that they are, and how must society and family relationships change in order to minimise the risk of the next generation taking the same path? And in saying that, I do not wish to imply that all young people have problems with alcohol, they do not, but the sad fact is that many do, and are at risk of doing serious damage to themselves and others before they hardly get a foot on the ladder into adulthood.

What of my relationship with Gary? Yes, it took a while to become established, I think. I had to resolve my own reactions in order to be as fully congruent as I could be. As it emerged what had happened in his past, I felt for him more and more. And could see the confusion that was going to emerge. It wasn't easy, as I say, but why should it be easy? Therapy is not easy, and counselling – and particularly working in a relational way as I do as a person-centred counsellor – is demanding and disciplined. But I know that if I can get the relationship right – well, maybe I should say get myself right in the relationship – I know that offering a constructive relational experience does promote constructive personality change.

Looking back, there were some powerful silences during the sessions. I often think silences are not given the attention they deserve. They are profound moments, or periods, of inter-communication between client and counsellor, but also, and sometimes more importantly, intra-communication within the client. Yet the counsellor remains present, maintaining a heartfelt and human presence which I believe does have an effect. However much a client becomes absorbed into what becomes present for them, they are no longer alone with it. There is another person bearing witness, validating the reality of what the client is going through. I do not think we understand the healing power of relationship.

It is often bad, difficult, abusive relational experiences that shape people in ways that cause them suffering and psychological distress and develop behaviours that can be destructive to themselves and others. We need to identify the components of what we might term "right relationship", and the power of the person-centred approach is that it does just that. Congruence – encompassing authenticity, realness, transparency, genuineness, and being present and integrated into relationship with the client; empathy – letting the client know that what they are saying and experiencing is being witnessed, heard, appreciated and to some degree understood; unconditional positive regard – warm acceptance, loving understanding, compassion, non-judgementalism, all encouraging the client to begin to genuinely offer themselves unconditional positive self-regard.

My work with Gary will continue for as long as he feels he wants to attend. During that time I will endeavour to offer the attitudinal qualities of the person-centred approach and I hope to watch him develop into a young man with greater self-awareness, a fuller appreciation of his choices, and a readiness to create for himself a lifestyle that satisfies his needs as a person increasingly liberated from the damaging effects of his past.'

An alternative outcome for Gary

Of course, Gary might not have taken up the offer of counselling, preferring to stay with his chosen behaviour, holding his anger and frustration locked up inside himself, his hatred for his father, his need to drink to explode in acts of violence. What might have been the outcome?

It was three weeks later, Gary was out drinking with his mates; they'd gone on to a club and it was 2.30 am. They left. It had been another evening of pent-up aggression. The music was loud, everything felt so intense. Gary knew he wanted to explode, knew he wanted to lay into someone, anyone, just looking, waiting, wound up ready to lash out.

The guy that had upset him had left. Lucky for him, Gary thought. Yeah, lucky for him. But he hadn't gone far. He was just around the corner, with his mates, waiting. They'd seen Gary before, the way he reacted, picked on people. He'd messed with one of their number before. They'd let it go, but he was a pain. He was still the same. They weren't going to have any more of it. No need to make a fuss in the club, no point in that. Fools picked fights in crowds. Want a serious fight, nice dark alley, no one to pull you off, no one to stop you. Yeah, they were going to teach him a lesson, one he wouldn't forget. They waited.

Gary was walking a little ahead as he turned into the darkened street behind the club. They jumped him, formed a circle and kicked him down to the ground. Mal and Luke were slow to react. They ran towards the group, three of them peeled off to face them. 'You want some as well, you fucked up shits?'

They hesitated. They could hear the thud of boots on bone and flesh. They hesitated, then ran. They weren't chased, the pack had their victim. It was only when they heard the commotion from the club that they realised that they must have alerted others. The pack retreated into the darkness. Gary was still breathing, just, but bleeding badly, with broken ribs, arms and ankle. His face was a mess. They'd stamped on his hands and feet. It wasn't clear whether he was going to survive . . .

PART 2

Carrie's story

'Drinking makes the feeling depressed worse?' Sally voiced her empathic response with a questioning tone, inviting Carrie to elaborate if she wished.

'Can do. It's best when I just, you know, pass out. I can get away from everything. I like that.'

'That feeling of getting away from it, you like that.'

Carrie nodded. She knew she was aware of knowing how at times she wished she was dead, but she didn't say anything. She felt anxious as she thought about it, her heart was thumping. She sniffed again and reached for another tissue as she felt more tears spilling over her eyelids. 'I wish everything was different.'

'If only, if only it could all be different.'

CHAPTER 7

Friday afternoon, 12 June

It was a hot afternoon and Carrie was glad to be away from the school. She hated the lessons, the teachers, everything. But it wasn't just school, it was her life that she hated, and herself. Everything was horrible and she had nowhere to escape to – until she started drinking, but that was a couple of years or more back and, yeah, it had brought her trouble. She'd been banned from school for drunkenness, but now she was back and, well, she'd sort of made an effort, sort of. But it was a hot, sunny day and she didn't want to stay near that school a moment longer.

She was with Maggs, and they'd pooled their money and got a bottle of vodka. It wasn't difficult. They knew one of the older lads in the sixth form, and he was happy to get it for them. Well, he liked to grope the girls and it was worth it to get the booze. They were now heading off to Maggs' house – no point in going to hers, her mother'd be drunk by now and she didn't like her friends coming round and seeing her.

Ten minutes later and they were up in Maggs' room, the stereo on and they passed the bottle back and forward between them. They didn't care about anything much, just liked the sensation of getting pissed. At least, Maggs liked the sensation, and so did Carrie, but in a different way. Carrie had things she wanted to forget, places in herself she wanted to keep away from. Maggs just liked the sensation of being drunk, feeling different, feeling good, that's how it felt for her.

They were both 15 and couldn't wait to get away. They were trying to get down to the school work, well, sometimes, but it didn't come easy to either of them. So much simpler to forget it all and sink into that lovely warm fuzziness.

Time passed and the bottle was emptied. In fact they fell asleep and awoke when they heard Maggs' mother come back. It was now 6.30 pm. They hadn't planned to still be there. They both stirred themselves, and they both felt very groggy. They looked at each other and giggled. They were still both very drunk.

'What're we gonna do, Maggs?'

'Oh, we'll just walk down the stairs and go out for a while. We'll feel better if we go out.'

'Or we could stay here, maybe she won't come in if we're quiet.'

They agreed to stay in the room and suppress their giggles.

Maggs' mum had had a heavy day at work and had called in at the supermarket on the way home. She had a lot of shopping to unload. She called out to Maggs, but there was no answer. No music, probably out somewhere. So she carried on bringing in the shopping and putting it away.

Upstairs the two girls had drifted back into a drunken sleep once more. They both felt really heavy, like their bodies just didn't want to move.

It was half an hour later when Maggs' mum came into the room. She'd finished downstairs and was just checking that the room was tidy. Both girls were asleep. She saw the empty vodka bottle in the corner, and shook her head. She blamed Carrie, she was bad news. She was sure she encouraged her daughter. Oh well, she thought, let them sleep it off. Maybe they'll learn when they wake up with bad heads. She decided to leave quietly and just wait to see how long it was before they woke up. She knew there was no point in calling Carrie's mother, she drank so much, and she was sure that was where Carrie got it from. She went back downstairs and started to cook the meal. Her husband was going to be late back – he was working away and wasn't expected back until late evening.

Carrie and Maggs are both starting out on their 'drinking careers'. Though drinking for different reasons, they are both already using alcohol problematically, and putting themselves at risk in bouts of intoxication. There's heavy alcohol use in Carrie's family and she's picked up the habit – for her own reasons, but nevertheless no doubt linked in some way to the way she has seen alcohol being used, and abused, for much of her life. Maggs has been drawn to alcohol for her own reasons – she simply likes the effect – but drinking to the degree that they both have is highly risky.

By leaving them to sleep it off, Maggs' mother has demonstrated she has no awareness of the risk of people vomiting after drinking heavily, and therefore putting their lives at risk. She has also assumed just the one bottle between them, but they may have drunk more, or used other substances as well. It highlights the need for education not only for young people with regard to the effects of alcohol use and abuse, but also for parents as well.

Friday evening

Carrie stirred later that evening, she hadn't been asleep, she'd passed out and she was lucky. She'd been sick but had fortunately been lying on her side and hadn't choked on the vomit. She felt awful. Maggs was still asleep.

'Maggs, Maggs, wake up, I've been sick.'

Maggs took a deep breath and rubbed her eyes, yawning as she did so.

'Shit, what's that smell?'

'I've been sick.'

'Oh shit!'

'Sorry.' Carrie got up, she still felt very unsteady.

'You'd better go and wash yourself in the bathroom.'

'Yeah, OK. What if your mum comes?'

'Just try and be quiet.'

Carrie rose unsteadily to her feet and moved towards the door. She was still feeling very disorientated as she opened it and went out on to the landing. She could smell food being cooked from the kitchen below, it made her feel sick. She hurried along to the bathroom. As she hurried to the toilet, she could feel herself wanting to be sick again, everything seemed to shift into slow motion. She'd caught her foot on the rug and at any other time, she'd have easily steadied herself, but she still had most of the contents of half a bottle of vodka inside her, and she lost her balance completely.

She felt herself falling and then a sharp thump on her shoulder. She tried to put her hands out to cushion her fall but fell on to the bathroom scales, her right arm caught under her body. She heard a snap and felt a sharp pain. She cried out.

Maggs ran, also somewhat unsteadily, from the bedroom and was joined by her mother who had heard the thump above and the cry – the bathroom was just above the kitchen.

'What's going on?'

'My arm, my arm . . .' was all Carrie could say.

Maggs' mother went over to her to see what had happened and tried to move her from where she had fallen. Carrie cried out in agony. 'Aaahh.'

'Maggs, stay with her, I'm calling an ambulance.' Her mother went into her own bedroom and dialed 999. No she couldn't bring her daughter's friend to the hospital, she was lying in agony on the bathroom floor and she couldn't move her.

'OK, there's an ambulance on its way. Carrie, can you get up?'

'I-I don't know. It hurts.'

'Can you roll over, off of the scales? Let me help you.' She stooped down and helped Carrie to move off her arm. She realised that Carrie had been sick where she had fallen.

'Vodka, huh?'

'We didn't mean to . . .'

'No, well, that's a conversation for another time. Maybe you'll both learn something from this.'

Carrie was in too much pain to feel anything for what she'd done. Her arm looked strange, like it was at a funny angle. She realised that her shoulder was hurting as well. She tried to move her neck but her shoulder became more painful.

'I think I hurt my shoulder as well.'

Maggs' mother hadn't noticed Carrie's shoulder; now as she looked she could see that it was clearly not looking right, maybe it was dislocated.

'You'd better just lie there, and Maggs, make yourself useful. Wipe up the sick, we might as well have the place a little cleaned up. Use that cloth.' She pointed to a cloth by the sink. Maggs did what she was asked, although till rather unsteadily.

'I'm sorry.' Carrie was speaking through her tears. Her arm didn't seem so painful but her shoulder was still hurting, in spite of the alcohol in her body. 'I-I was sick in the bedroom as well.'

Maggs' mother shook her head and closed her eyes. 'Well, you can sort that out when you've finished in here, Maggs. I'll go downstairs and turn the cooker off. You stay here and do something useful.' She looked at her daughter as she spoke.

'I'm sorry, Maggs.'

'It's OK, it must be awful.'

Carrie couldn't nod her head without moving her shoulder. She winced as she tried.

Maggs carried on clearing up. A couple of minutes later and her mother had returned.

'Right, I'd better call your parents, Carrie, they need to know what's happened here. I presume you drank that bottle of vodka I saw empty in the bedroom earlier?'

Maggs nodded.

'OK, well, what's their number, Carrie?' Maggs had the cordless phone with her. Carrie gave her the number.

'Hello? Is that Carrie's mother?'

The voice said yes, though with a definite slur.

'I'm Maggie's mother, Carrie's friend. Look, Carrie's fallen over and damaged her arm. I've called for an ambulance and they've said they'll be here very soon.'

'What's she been doing now?'

'Drinking.' She restrained herself from saying, 'like you'. 'Anyway, that's beside the point. She needs medical attention and I guess she'll be going to the local hospital. I'll call to let you know.'

'I'll tell her father. We'd better come over.'

The door bell rang. 'I think the ambulance has arrived. I'll just check.'

She went downstairs, taking the phone with her. She explained what had happened and checked where they would be taking Carrie. She gave the information to Carrie's mother, who agreed they'd best go straight to the hospital.

Counselling session 1: silence as the therapeutic process begins

Thursday 18 June

Sally sat opposite the young girl that had come into the counselling room. She seemed very withdrawn, and quite pale. That wasn't unusual. She saw people of all ages. Working at the accident and emergency department as an alcohol counsellor meant that she had a constant flow of clients. Not all experienced their alcohol use as a problem, though it often was.

For many younger binge drinkers the initial problem may be identified from outside the health services: within the family, at school, at a youth club, for instance. In all of these cases it is important for information to be available for those who identify that the young person has, or may have, a problem with alcohol, and that they know who they can encourage the young person to see, or who they might get information and advice from themselves. Often the young person will listen to someone they already have a relationship with, someone they respect, rather than bringing in another person.

One difficulty can lie in how much pressure is exerted on a young person to attend a service, whoever is providing it. Too much pressure can be negative, encouraging resistance. At any age it is difficult to acknowledge a problem with alcohol, but if greater openness can be encouraged generally within the social world of the young people about the potentially damaging and problematic effects of binge drinking, then there is likely to be scope for more open discussion with the young person who is exhibiting signs of difficulty.

Often peer education can be helpful. This can take the form of projects within schools or at youth centres. There are also theatrical groups that present on alcohol- and drug-related themes to encourage debate, and to raise awareness. Information about alcohol and its effects needs to be made more widely available throughout society and particularly within all services who work directly with young people, whatever the context.

She smiled across at the young girl, who had glanced up. She didn't smile back, but looked away again. Carrie hated herself, didn't want to be there. It was only because the doctor and the nurse had insisted that she came back to see this counsellor. She didn't want to talk to anyone, just wanted to get on with her life. Yeah, she thought, just get on with my life. She then thought about how much she hated her life, her parents, their drinking. But theirs was different. She drank because it was cool, yeah, what she liked to do with her mates, particularly Maggs. Yeah, OK, so she'd been unlucky, broke her arm. Well, so what. Bit of a laugh really, didn't know quite what all the fuss had been about. So she'd got pissed. She wasn't the only one, she was just unlucky, probably wouldn't happen again. But everyone else seemed concerned and told her she had to talk about her drinking. What was there to talk about? She sat, staring at a poster on the wall, though not really paying it much attention. She heard the counsellor speaking to her.

'So, I know you had an accident, broke your arm, and the nurse wanted you to come and have a chat to me about your drinking.'

Carrie continued to stare. She didn't want to be there. Had enough of hospitals, horrible places. She heard the news, you got bugs in them, people died, she didn't want any of that.

Sally could see that Carrie clearly didn't want to be there, and the idea of communicating to her anything about the nature of counselling wasn't going to be easy. She knew that the nurse had given Carrie an information leaflet, and she was grateful for that. Whether she had read it, well, that was another matter. But that could wait. What was important was for her, as the counsellor, to offer the therapeutic conditions to create the opportunity for a therapeutic relationship to develop.

The person-centred approach as we have seen emphasises the therapeutic relationship. While there may be a need for assessments, agreed and informed consent, the reality is that before anything of that nature can happen, communication has to be taking place between client and counsellor. A relationship has to be being formed. Where the person-centred approach differs from other approaches is the primacy that it gives to building the therapeutic relationship. While some might argue that there has to be consent for treatment, or there has to be an in-depth assessment before counselling can start, this is not a person-centred perspective. Yes, these may take place, but they can also be a barrier if introduced inappropriately to relationship building.

Sally had decided to respond to what Carrie was communicating, which seemed to be a lack of interest in being there. Yes, she realised it was her interpretation, and she would own that, but she also felt it was vitally important to be open and upfront, particularly, she found, with younger people. At least, that was her experience.

'Seems to me, and I may be wrong, but it seems to me that you really don't want to be here.'

Carrie took a deep breath and sighed. 'No,' she thought to herself, 'I don't.' She didn't say anything.

Sally heard the sigh. 'Seems to me that you're here because someone else wants you to be here. Or have I got that wrong?'

Carrie found herself shaking her head. Still looking at the poster. She suddenly turned to look at Sally. 'I've got nothing to say.'

'Mhmm, there's nothing you really want to talk about.' She smiled and nodded slightly as she spoke, maintaining the eye contact.

Carrie shrugged and turned to look away again.

Sally remained calm. She wasn't going to rush in and push Carrie into saying anything she didn't want to. She could see tension in Carrie's body, the way she was sitting. She seemed quite stiff, tense. And she still had her arm in a sling.

Carrie turned to Sally again. 'They kept having a go, telling me I had a problem. Well I haven't. So I fell over, so what?'

'Yeah, so let me check I've got this right, it feels like they had a go, but for you, you just fell over, not a problem.' Sally sought to convey her understanding of what Carrie was saying. She was not offering a reflection which is something else, although the words can appear the same. She was coming from a place of trying to understand and be clear that she was understanding exactly what Carrie was saying.

'You going to tell me I've got a problem?'

'Is that what you're expecting?'

'S'ppose so.'

'Mhmm. Well, no, I'm not, I don't work that way.'

Carrie frowned, unsure, uncertain of what to make of what had just been said. 'So what do you do?'

'I listen, I try to understand what people are experiencing and telling me.'

'That all?'

'Not everyone feels listened to in their lives, or feels anyone is trying to understand them.' Sally responded as she saw her role and why it was so important. So many people seemed to think there was nothing to listening, to empathising, but Sally knew different, knew it was a focused and disciplined way of being towards another person.

This is an interesting response, an attempt perhaps to relate to what may be the client's experience. It is also very true. And there is a belief that it's easy to listen and empathise, but the person-centred approach affirms the importance of how you listen and the nature of how you respond. It is not a matter of simply reflecting back what someone has said in order for them to feel heard. Is it enough to merely hear your own words to genuinely feel heard, really feel heard? It is also a matter of tone of voice, facial expression, posture, and also what is being experienced by the counsellor towards their client. Is warm acceptance present? Is the counsellor accurately present and genuine in what they are feeling, thinking and communicating?

It cannot be too strongly emphasised that the person-centred approach is not about telling the client what they have just told you. All that needs is a good memory. Clients don't want a memory in the chair opposite them, they want a person, a human being who can, indeed we should say who genuinely wants to, form a person-to-person relationship based on respect, unconditional positive regard, and a striving for authenticity, congruence, transparency.

Carrie sighed again. That was true. No one really listened to her, not really listened. In a way that was good – sometimes. She could do her own stuff, her parents didn't seem too bothered. She sort of wanted them to listen, sometimes, but, well, they didn't, just had a go, on her case. She shook her head.

'Leaves you shaking your head, yeah?'

'People don't listen, do they? Not really. They just want to tell you all the time, "do this, don't do that". But they don't listen, not really. Your mates do, your real mates, yeah, they'll listen, you know, when you're serious, yeah, real mates will . . .' Carrie paused, thinking of some of the heart-to-hearts that she and Maggs had had. They were good mates, really good mates, though since the accident . . . , she wasn't sure, seemed like Maggs was sort of different, well, not so much different, but sort of a bit distant somehow. She didn't understand it.

'So, people don't listen to you, except your mates, not seriously listen anyway.'

Carrie stared ahead of herself, she heard the words but somehow they didn't really make an impression. Her shoulder still felt tender, as did her arm. She thought back to the accident and emergency department, to the nurse who had asked her all those questions about her drinking. She'd answered, let her fill in her form, but then she'd said about wanting her to come back to see the counsellor.

Specialist responses to people presenting with alcohol-related problems at accident and emergency departments have been established in some hospitals. The idea is to broach the topic while the negative effects of alcohol use are clearly present and often visible. Different hospitals take different approaches. Often a questionnaire is used to quickly ascertain the amount of drinking occurring. It could be a specialist nurse receiving referrals, it could be accident and emergency staff trained up in brief interventions and motivational interviewing techniques, it could be a counsellor offering regular sessions for patients identified as having an alcohol issue that could be usefully explored. The case for some form of response within accident and emergency departments is very strong.

She continued to sit, saying nothing. Still, she thought, at least being here, if she kept coming, would mean time not at school. She was going back next week, but maybe this was a good reason to have some time away. That was something. She smiled slightly at the thought.

Sally noticed the smile and responded to it. 'Makes you smile?'

Carrie nodded but didn't respond. The smile dropped away from her face. 'Nothing.'

'OK.' Sally could sense that clearly Carrie wasn't going to say anything more about it, and she respected that and accepted it.

Carrie felt slightly surprised that Sally hadn't pushed her. That was what adults did, asked questions, wanted to know all the time. Well, some did, her dad did, teachers did, the doctor and the nurse did, her mum did sometimes as well. Always questions and people telling her what she should do, what she should think, at school, at home. Why couldn't people get off her case? She wanted to be left alone. Yeah, that's what she wanted, not on her own, but with her mates, messing around, having a laugh, winding the boys up.

Sally fully accepted Carrie not wanting to say any more. She noticed the smile returning to Carrie's face but she did not respond to it this time. Carrie wasn't giving her eye contact, though Sally was available for that. She didn't sit staring at Carrie. She'd look away and then return to looking over to Carrie's face.

An interesting issue. How much eye contact does a counsellor give to a client, or at least how much do they look towards the client's face when a client is clearly not wanting to return eye contact? What is an empathic response in this situation? How does the counsellor convey warm acceptance of the client? Does it make a difference that the client is a young person? Having someone continually looking at you is likely to make people feel uncomfortable in a situation that is probably unusual to them anyway. There has to be a balance somehow, between maintaining availability for eye contact, maintaining an awareness of the client's facial expression, but without just continually looking at them throughout a prolonged silence.

Sally knew she didn't know precisely why Carrie was choosing not to speak. She did not know her well enough to understand her reasons. But she appreciated that not everyone wanted to talk, to disclose things about themselves. While she knew that in many areas of counselling there was a demand for an assessment, for questions to be asked and answered, this was not her approach, and not the way she wanted to start to establish a relationship with her clients. Indeed, she felt at times that it could be anti-therapeutic. Yet she also recognised that there was a place for this in certain settings, where perhaps information was needed to help someone who was at risk of harm, say. But often they were situations that were not purely counselling ones. Questions had been asked of her client and, as a result, Carrie had been referred to her. Now it was for her to form a therapeutic relationship with Carrie and offer her the opportunity to experience an unconditionally accepting relationship, probably a new experience for her as it was for most people, yet an opportunity for her to risk being open to herself in a relational climate of transparency and authenticity. Yes, Sally thought, the picture of what is happening for Carrie will emerge over time. She felt sure Carrie would tell her what she wanted to have heard when she felt ready to do so.

Carrie wasn't prepared to accept her drinking as being a problem. Yes, her mother had a problem, she knew she drank too much, but that was her. She, Carrie, was different. Just a laugh, get off your face, yeah, good feeling. She felt good, like everything could be sort of forgotten, nothing sort of mattered. She liked that. It was a good, positive experience. OK, so she'd fallen over, but that was an accident. Nothing more than that. And, yeah, she'd been sick, so what, it happened. The nurse had told her that it was risky, she could have died. Carrie had sort of heard her but, well, she hadn't, had she? What did the nurse know? She didn't want to think about it any more.

A person who passes out under the influence of alcohol is at very real risk of death from asphyxiation if they vomit, particularly if they are lying on their back and the vomit cannot drain out of the mouth. The suppressant effect of the alcohol can also inhibit the breathing reflex, which heightens the risk. The nurse was right to point this out. Anyone who passes out from alcohol, or for any reason, needs to be placed into the recovery position if that is possible.

Sally was aware of a sense that the silence was feeling a little more tense. Was it her? Was she finding it difficult? Or was she picking up on discomfort in Carrie? She didn't feel tense, and yet there was a kind of unease. Her thoughts turned to what Carrie had said about people not listening. She wondered if, given that was her experience, whether it left Carrie feeling less able, or less willing, to talk when someone was listening, except for her mates. She could imagine how if, over time, you had that sense of no one really wanting to listen to what you had to say, that you might begin to think that you weren't worth listening to. A kind of condition of worth would arise. Or rather, a condition of lack of worth. And then what could emerge might be the thought that, well, if I'm not going to be listened to I'd best learn to feel good about not being listened to, and so I'll say things or behave in ways that reinforce that. It may not be a conscious process, but it could happen.

At this point Sally found herself slipping into wondering how Carrie, as a 15-year-old girl, was experiencing being with her, a 38-year-old counsellor.

She brought her thoughts back to the present, taking in Carrie's expression and her body language. She seemed slumped in the chair. She'd looked down and was picking at her nails. She knew that she accepted Carrie's need to be as she needed to be, and somehow, in that moment, she felt a particular warmth for her. She suddenly seemed to Sally to look somehow separate, cut off in some way. It was quite an intense experience, and then it passed. She felt she needed to communicate something to Carrie, something of her own presence, of her own feeling for her. She knew that for her empathy, unconditional positive regard and authenticity to have therapeutic value, well, they had to be experienced as being present by the client. That was what she believed, anyway. No good her sitting there with all those 'core conditions' and none of them reaching the client.

Carrie continued to sit, picking at her nails, lost in a kind of blankness. She wasn't really thinking about anything. Her arms felt heavy, the plaster was a pain sometimes. Still, she'd got some great messages on it. The one thought she did have was around people on her case all the time, she wanted some space, her space, to do what she wanted.

Sally's thoughts, meanwhile, had turned back to something Carrie had said earlier and which Sally was suddenly aware of feeling that she had not responded to. Yes, Carrie had spoken about not feeling listened to and, yes, she'd responded to that. And then the silence. Was there something she wasn't hearing, hadn't heard? There had been something else. And she realised that she hadn't shown empathy for that. Hmm, why? She remembered what it was and, yes, it felt like a supervision issue. But that was for later.

'It may not be what you're thinking about now, but I'm thinking about what you said about people not just not listening, but also how they tell you what to do, "do this, don't do that". I wanted you to know that I did hear that although I didn't respond to it at the time. Yeah, must really piss you off.'

Carrie felt herself frown, not sure how to react to what had been said. She was slightly taken aback and yet somehow it sort of felt good hearing it. Sort of sounded like she meant it. She shrugged and picked at her nails a little more intently.

'Things you perhaps want to tell them but they just don't want to hear.' Sally felt that her words sort of resonated with the moment in some way. She knew that didn't sound too scientific, but they flowed out of her mouth, they sort of felt right, somehow. She'd learnt to trust these kinds of experiences. Although she hadn't on the face of it got much contact with Carrie, and yet somehow she did feel such a strong sense of Carrie's presence, and that sense of her feeling cut off was back, like she needed to be reached out to. But was that her need, or Carrie's, or a figment of her over-active, over-sensitive, imagination?

Counsellors can experience strong feelings, urges, to speak and say particular things. But they do need to be weighed up. Does what has emerged feel like it has relevance to the therapeutic relationship? Is now the time to voice it? Should I let it go and then only voice it later if it persists and still feels relevant? How does the counsellor know (judge?) what is relevant anyway? The person-centred counsellor seeks to stay within the frame of reference of the client, but there are experiences that emerge into the counsellor's awareness that seem to be connected to the relational process, however minimal that might be.

'I want them all to leave me alone.'

'Leave you alone . . .'

'Yeah, just let me get on with my life, you know?'

'Mhmm, that just sounds so important for you to feel left alone to get on with your life.' Sally spoke softly but clearly, wanting to convey that she was hearing what Carrie was saying, but not to leave Carrie listening to what she had said and taking her away from the flow of experiencing that was present for her, within her.

'Always having a go.' Carrie shook her head, she was still looking down. She continued to pick at her nails. The fore finger of her broken right arm was getting most of the attention.

'That's how it feels, people always having a go at you.' Sally nodded slightly.

'Why can't they leave me alone?' Carrie suddenly looked up. There was anger in her voice, her jaw seemed set hard, her eyes blazed.

'Why? Why can't they leave you alone?' Sally matched Carrie's tone of voice.

'They don't understand, none of them do.'

'Mhmm, they just don't understand what it is like for you.' Sally felt so genuine in her responses, she had a really strong sense of how much Carrie hated how everyone was towards her.

Carrie didn't want to say anything more. She felt angry, sad, ashamed, and hateful. She wanted to say things, but bit them back. The shame blocked her from saying more.

Carrie was shaking her head and looking down again. 'But I ain't got a problem.'

'No, no, I hear you, it's not a problem.'

The way Carrie heard Sally made her feel suddenly very, very sad. She swallowed, her throat felt raw all of a sudden, and it felt like it had a huge hot, heavy lump in it. She forced her feeling back, she wasn't going to let anyone see. She coped, she was good at coping, not like her mum. She couldn't cope with anything, just drank, just got pissed all the time. And her dad seemed to put up with it, and that pissed her off as well. He didn't seem to care. They'd row sometimes, yeah, who didn't, but never violent, nothing like that. Shouting and door slamming. Been like that for a while. He'd drink as well, but later, in the evenings. She was usually asleep by then. She didn't know why they were together although she kind of thought it was for her. For her! What was there for her? She was shaking her head, her jaw was tight, the sadness replaced by anger once more, but also there was still the shame, the shame of having crap parents. Yeah, her mates moaned about theirs but, well, what did they know? But she didn't really want them to know, though some of them did. But she'd defend them, they were her parents, she hated them, but deep down, almost out of sight, she so wanted to feel that they loved her.

Carrie felt like she'd had enough. 'Can I go now?'

'Is that what you want?'

Carrie shrugged. 'You gonna want to see me again?'

'I'd like to give you some more time. It can take a while getting used to counselling, having time to talk, having someone listen to you and not tell you what to do all the time.'

'Yeah, that sounds good. You don't, do you, you just listen.'

'Mhmm, yeah, that's what I do.'

'Weird.'

'Feels weird?'

'Yeah, I mean, people don't do they, you know, not like this.'

'No, this is different.'

'So, when do I come back?'

'Next week?' Sally didn't want to lose any momentum in the relationship building process.

Carrie nodded.

'I'll give you an appointment card, and I'll sign it. Same time, same day?'

'OK.'

'So, it felt weird, yeah?'

'You do sort of listen but that's ... I mean, I don't know what to talk about. And, well, I don't have a problem.'

'I know, it really doesn't seem like a problem.'

'I can handle it.'

'Handle ... ?'

'Drinking, you know?'

'Mhmm, drinking isn't a problem, you can handle it.'

'What happened was unlucky.'

Sally was very aware that having thought the session was ending it now felt as though it had started again, and once more back to Carrie vociferously affirming that she didn't have a problem with her drinking. It was obvious to Sally that this was something that it was really important for Carrie to believe and to convince herself of.

'Mhmm, just unlucky, an unfortunate accident.'

Carrie knew she didn't want it to be like that again. It had really hurt, but she felt sure it wouldn't happen again. She wasn't like her mum, just having a few laughs. Yeah, having a few drinks felt good. Surely this counsellor would understand that? 'Everyone drinks, you know, makes you feel good.'

'A way to feel good, something everyone does.'

'I was unlucky.'

'Mhmm. So you're not going to let it happen again?'

'No, I mean, yeah, I'll still, you know, get pissed and that, but not do that again.'

'Still get pissed but, yeah, not fall over and break your arm another time.'

'No.' Carrie shook her head. 'No.'

'Mhmm, you sound pretty clear about all of that, Carrie, you'll get pissed again, but you won't fall over and won't break your arm again. You sound really sure about that.'

'That's right. Haven't had a drink since, you know, but I will.'

'Mhmm, it sort of sounds like that's really important, or maybe I'm not getting that right.'

'Yeah, yeah, it is. I want to have a few laughs, you know, makes you feel good.'

'Mhmm, makes you feel good, have a few laughs, just don't fall over, yeah?'

'Nurse told me to control it, stop getting pissed, would put me at risk. I know that, you know, I can handle it.'

'Not something you wanted to hear because you know you can handle it?'

'I don't like people telling me what I can and can't do, yeah?'

'Mhmm, sure, and didn't like hearing someone tell you to stop getting pissed, that it would put you at risk.'

'No, no.'

'Mhmm.'

During this last piece of dialogue there could be a tension, it depends on the counsellor's tone of voice. Is she really accepting what her client is saying and feeling about her alcohol use? Yes, there is empathic responding, but is there warm acceptance? The counsellor could be at risk of not offering the therapeutic conditions with what then occurs being less therapeutically helpful, particularly at such an early stage in the counselling process where there is a need for the client to genuinely feel heard as part of the relationship-building process. The client can be left feeling judged, and not necessarily consciously. It could be an experience that is not fully present in awareness, a kind of psychological reflex in response to a sense that the counsellor may not be fully accepting of the client's perception of their reality. The counsellor may not be sufficiently sensitive to the fact that this is what is happening. Hence the need for continued supervision and personal development to ensure that the counsellor's awareness is sufficiently open to their own experiencing.

The session was due to end and Sally checked out how Carrie felt, and pointed out that people could feel a bit odd after counselling, that it could be quite intense, a lot of thinking and feeling and concentrating. 'You might want to take it carefully, can feel a bit overwhelming when you get back outside sometimes, or some people feel so absorbed in what they are thinking or feeling that they forget to think about what they are doing, like crossing the road. So, you know, take care, take it easy.'

Carrie nodded. She appreciated that. It felt genuine. Someone who, yeah, seemed to care. She didn't really think about it so much as being aware that it sort of made an impression upon her. She couldn't quite define it, not that she was trying, but it did make an impression. It left Carrie a little more thoughtful when she left and headed off to get the bus home. She'd decided to phone Maggs, hadn't seen much of her being off school for a few days. Maggs hadn't phoned.

Points for discussion

- Assess Sally's application of person-centred principles in this opening counselling session.
- What is your reaction to Sally's thoughts about assessment? In what situation might a formal assessment be necessary? Contrast these settings with the nature and purpose of person-centred counselling.
- How might you have responded to Carrie's silence? Would you have said more, less, and why?
- Why do you think Carrie started talking more fluidly towards the end of the session? What do you think might have been her internal process, seen from a person-centred theoretical perspective?
- What would you take to supervision from this session?

Write notes for this session.

CHAPTER 8

Counselling session 2: silence, distance and then the client discloses more

Thursday 25 June

Carrie sat in the waiting area. She felt good to have a reason not to be at school. She was thinking as well about the previous week, what it had been like seeing a counsellor. Weird, she thought. She still wasn't too sure about it. Felt like she had done a lot of, well, sitting. And yet ... ? It had been weird but it had also been kind of different in a sort of ... , she wasn't sure how to describe it. Sally was different, at least she seemed somehow different, not quite like other people, somehow, not really what she had expected. Not really. She had felt sure there'd be lots of questions and lots of being told what she must and mustn't do. But there hadn't been any of that at all. And that felt sort of good, somehow, but strange as well.

She'd wondered if that was all counselling was. If so, she felt she could cope with that. Yes, she thought, as she sat there waiting for her appointment time, she could cope with that. After all, that's what she did best, most of the time anyway, cope with all the crap in her life.

Carrie's thoughts drifted back to the previous evening, another furious row at home between her parents. She hated it, hated them, hated being there, and at times hated herself. She blamed them both; her mother for drinking so much and in the way that she did, her father for not dealing with it, with her, and then often ending the evening drinking himself and just being, well, so bloody miserable all of the time.

She heard her name and looked up, her train of thought fading as she saw Sally.

'Hi Carrie, ready to come through?'

Carrie nodded and got up, following Sally towards the counselling room. She went in and sat in the chair she had sat in the previous week.

'How's the arm?'

'A little better, more awkward than anything else. I'm back at school though now.' She spoke the last bit without much enthusiasm.

'You don't seem too pleased about the being back at school part.'

'Don't like it, don't see the point, not really. But you have to, you know? I want to leave as soon as I can, get a job, get some money, have some fun.'

'Mhmm, leave, job, money and fun.' Sally nodded as she spoke. What Carrie had said seemed pretty clear.

'You've got to, haven't you. Well, I have to anyway.' Carrie was thinking of wanting to get away from home as well, though she knew it would take her a while to be able to afford that. But maybe, one day, she knew she would. She knew she had to. She couldn't wait. And, well, it also made her sad, but she didn't want to feel that now and she pushed the feelings away. She wasn't always able to do that, but this time she did.

'Having fun sounds really, really important to you.' Sally felt thoroughly genuine in her response. It felt very clear given not only what Carrie had said, but the way she had said it.

'Things get you down, you know? Need a few laughs, makes you feel good.'

'Mhmm, have some fun and a few laughs.' Sally nodded, 'it's good to feel good.'

Carrie nodded, suddenly also very aware of the contrast in herself, that she also spent a lot of time not feeling good. She went silent, not only in terms of stopping speaking, but inside herself as well.

It seemed to Sally that Carrie had suddenly withdrawn from her, something had changed, as if she had pulled back, distanced herself in some way. Sally quickly checked herself. Was it her pulling back for some reason? She didn't think so. She didn't feel as though she had changed her focus in any way, just this sudden sense of distance. 'I don't know if this is your experience, but it feels like something has made you feel distant to me.' Sally chose to voice her experience rather than keep it to herself. Somehow her words sounded a bit awkward, didn't seem so clear and straight as she had hoped. But the moment had passed, she had said what she had said as an expression of what she was feeling. It had felt appropriate to say something.

> When does a counsellor disclose something that has emerged into their own awareness? Professional judgement is called for. Is the something sensed relevant to the therapeutic process? Does the counsellor, at the moment of its emergence, feel they are connected and very much integrated into the relationship with the client, or have they drifted into some other area of their own and what has emerged is more associated with that? Congruence, authenticity, transparency do not call for an endless stream of self-disclosure. Rather, they are concerned with making visible experiencing that emerges in response to the therapeutic process. A certain self-discipline is called for. Decisions have to be made very quickly. Often the fact that something persists in the counsellor's awareness can indicate that it is pressing and appropriate to voice, but again, as mentioned above, there should still be a consideration as to whether it is emerging from a sense of connection with the client.

Carrie felt very anxious, all of a sudden. She didn't know why. It was there, and she wanted to say something, but didn't want to as well, and both at the same time. Her heart was suddenly thumping. She didn't like it. She felt hot suddenly as well. She tightened her lips, it was an instinctive reaction, not wanting to let any words out. But she wanted to say something, although she didn't know what.

Sally remained aware of the sense of distance, like a gap had opened up, yet she wanted to reach across it, or at least maintain her presence in such a way that she was communicating her availability to Carrie, her availability as a person wanting to offer the possibility of a therapeutic relationship with her client. She felt a sense of caring and concern for Carrie. The change, the shift, had felt so sudden. One moment Carrie had been talking freely about wanting some fun, having a laugh, feeling good, and it felt like, yes, they were interacting quite freely. And then it was as though something had sort of pulled her back; or like a cloud or a veil or something had sort of passed between them. She was tempted to head down a speculative route with her thoughts, but brought herself away from it to focus herself on Carrie, on what was present, and being with that rather than getting caught into thinking about and analysing it. But what remained very present for her was the sense of the suddenness with which everything had changed.

The silence continued. Yet inwardly Carrie was not silent. The anxiety remained very present. She remained tight-lipped. She wanted to say how hateful things were, how she wished everything could be different, how she wanted to feel happy more of the time. At least, that's what she had initially felt, but the urgency had somehow faded a little. Her mood was dropping. Her heart wasn't thumping to quite the same degree, the anxiety was easing. It all just felt heavy and dark.

Incongruence is present in the client who is not denying her feelings to her awareness, but denying them in the sense of not allowing them to be made visible through communication. We can think of congruence in terms of organismic experience, awareness and communication, a triangular relationship. Where what is being experienced within the person is also accurately present in awareness, and that awareness can be accurately expressed in communication, then the person is in a more congruent state. Where there are blocks and distortions to this process then incongruence is present (Bryant-Jefferies, 2000).

Alcohol can add to the incongruence, distorting the person's awareness of what is being experienced, and how they interpret it. It also disrupts the flow between awareness and what is communicated, the person perhaps not being able to find the right words to express themselves accurately. Yet, it also has to be acknowledged that there will be times when alcohol enhances congruence, enabling, say, a part of the person that is usually silent to find its voice as a result of alcohol's disinhibiting influence.

In the dialogue, the client is aware of what they are experiencing, but they are not allowing themselves to express it. One way to think of this is to see the person as made up of parts, and one part which does not want the difficult feelings to be made visible, perhaps it is a part that feels shame at what they are feeling, maintains a constraining influence over the part that wants the hurt, in this case the feelings of hatefulness, to emerge into communication to the counsellor.

As a result of feelings not being voiced, the client's mood begins to drop. This could be the result of feeling drained by the internal battle that has taken place, it could be an internal reaction to not being able to say what is present, or it could be a straightforward symptom of incongruence.

The person-centred counsellor will seek to offer all aspects or parts of the client the same therapeutic qualities, recognising that all of the person needs to feel heard, understood, listened to, and warmly accepted in a spirit of openness.

Carrie continued to sit staring ahead of her, lost in her thoughts yet without really thinking. What was the point – that was the predominant thought, and yet it wasn't just in her head. It was more a sort of feeling than a thought, and it sort of pervaded her whole being. She sighed.

Sally heard the sigh and noticed a change in Carrie's expression. It was as though the brightness that had been present had faded. She looked sort of dulled in some way, yes, like the shine had been taken away. And yet it felt more than that. And it had again happened so quickly. Was this a kind of teenage process? And who was she to label it up in that way? Did it matter? What really mattered was that here was a 15-year-old girl suddenly going very quiet and distant, and who was suddenly looking like a light had gone out – was that too dramatic? A sudden switch. A symptom of something else? She felt herself breathing out. She hadn't realised that she had been holding it in. She realised that the tension of the moment had got into her own body. She felt on edge, suddenly very sensitive herself, feeling a need to be fine-tuned and responsive to Carrie.

Sally was aware that Carrie hadn't said much about herself and what her life was like. And she firmly believed in trusting her clients' inner processes; that they could and would share and explore what they needed to explore when they felt able to, or when their inner process demanded it of them in such a way that they were unable to restrain it. She believed that the presence of the therapeutic conditions encouraged . . . , was that the right word? Or was it enabled, or maybe facilitated, but whichever, the result was that the client could allow themselves to break through emotional and psychological barriers that might be present within them. It was a sensitive time, and a testing time in many ways. Could she, Sally, be the warm and accepting person, open and sensitive and fully present – or as fully present as she could be – in relationship with her client, whatever inner processes were emerging within her client and being expressed? She also felt herself wondering briefly what role alcohol might be playing in what Carrie experienced in herself, or in her way of managing this.

Alcohol does affect mood. It can disinhibit to begin with but after a couple of drinks the suppressant effect can begin to override the disinhibiting effect. Mood is more likely to then dip. Of course, context also plays a part. In a lively, social gathering, alcohol can enhance the experience. But for the person drinking alone, it can be a very different experience. For some people, mood can dip sharply, perhaps because they already have a tendency towards lower mood, or perhaps the alcohol opens the person's awareness to emotional and psychological material that is present within them that is simply depressing by its nature. Alcohol use is associated with suicidal idea-tion for some people, and actual suicide. People can feel a need to self-harm under the influence of alcohol, which can be more problematic as they may have less control over what they are doing, and be less cognisant of the risks.

Carrie felt in a familiar place in herself, all too familiar. She was used to it, but that didn't mean she liked it. More often than not, though, when she was feeling the way she was feeling now she wasn't really thinking about how she felt, she was simply being how she felt. It was overwhelming. She was what she felt and there was no psychological space within her awareness of any sense of being able to step aside from the feelings and reflect on them. The silence continued.

Sally did not want to break the silence, but at the same time she was concerned as to how much contact or psychological contact Carrie might be experiencing, and was aware that contact was a 'necessary condition for constructive psy-chological change' in terms of her approach to working with clients.

Carrie's mood remained low. When she felt this way she simply felt as though she was lost in some way, like feeling trapped in a heavy black fog. She could never make herself feel different. Sometimes something external could shift it, though often it seemed to gradually lift after a while. She was also aware that drinking sometimes made it a little easier, but it could make it worse as well. If she drank a lot, though, she could pass out and that was a release and a relief. She liked to feel herself heading for that kind of oblivion. She rarely spoke to anyone about it, it was what she did, how she coped. She hated it all as well and there were times when she wondered if she would be better off dead. And yet at other times that was so far away from her thinking and how she felt.

Sally felt it was time to make a verbal comment to at least remind Carrie that she was there for her. 'I'm wondering if there is anything you feel like saying. I'd like to hear if there is.' She spoke gently, wanting her words to feel like the offer they were, and not a demand. She was feeling concerned now, there was something heavy about the silence that had developed between them and it didn't feel healthy. It felt sort of stifling. She realised that what she was feeling was wholly subjective, Carrie had said nothing about how she felt, she was relying entirely on her own inner experiencing, but over the years as a counsellor, and as a person, she had grown to trust that more and more. The feelings she had now were very present for her, and they urged her to reach out.

Carrie responded by shaking her head, very slowly. It all felt an effort. And her arm and shoulder were aching and it all felt too much. And her parents, the row last night, there'd be a bad silence at home again and she really didn't want to experience that again. She knew she'd just go to her room. She often didn't want to go out when she felt like this. She wished she felt different, but just thinking about that seemed to be too much of an effort.

'Bad place, huh?' Again, Sally spoke softly, feeling assured that what she was saying was empathically accurate to what was happening.

Carrie nodded.

'Go there a lot?'

Carrie nodded again.

Sally nodded back. 'Anything I can do?' She spoke warmly and with a heartfelt genuineness in her concern and her desire to offer something.

Carrie felt a sense of Sally wanting to help. That was new. No one tried to help when she was like this. Her parents tended to ignore her, or tell her to liven herself up a bit. They never seemed very sympathetic, felt like they didn't want to know; felt like they didn't want to know her. It was a horrible feeling and sometimes it would make her angry, as well as sad. But the truth was she didn't know what she wanted, not in her awareness anyway. But deep down within her organismic experiencing, yet beyond the edge of her awareness, there existed a desperate cry to feel loved, understood, cared about. Carrie wanted to respond to Sally, but she didn't know what to say, and she was frightened as to what might happen if she did start to tell her anything about what was happening for her.

Carrie looked up and into the eyes of Sally. Sally on her part could feel waves of emotion inside herself, Carrie looked so desperate and suddenly so very vulnerable. 'Hard to know where to begin?'

Carrie nodded again, but this time she felt her throat feeling blocked, a heavy hot lump in her throat. She swallowed, it didn't shift it, and she felt tears welling up in her eyes. She tried to control them, tried to take a deep breath, but it was suddenly all too much. It was the expression on Sally's face, her eyes, she felt she could trust her, not something she was consciously thinking or being aware of, but something that existed at some more instinctive level.

> The impact of the therapeutic relationship may not always be consciously recognised. Sometimes the person can be affected at some deeper level like this, triggering the release of feeling or some form of expression that otherwise might have been restrained.

The tears streamed down Carrie's face. Sally nudged the box of tissues that were on the table towards her. Carrie took one and buried her face in it. 'I-I don't know what to say.'

'No, it's not always easy to find the words or know where to begin.'

'Both.'

'Yeah.' Sally nodded and reached over and gently squeezed Carrie's good arm. Sometimes when the words couldn't be found, then another way of conveying warmth and empathy for what a client was experiencing needed to be found. 'There's no rush, take your time, take all the time you need.' Sally knew that Carrie, as with any client, needed to take things at her own pace. She was now acknowledging that there were things she wanted to say and that it was all very upsetting for her. Sally was also aware that over half the session had passed, but she didn't have any other clients that day and felt OK if the session needed to overrun a bit. But she'd check that out later, if it came to that. For now, all that mattered was that she maintained her end of the therapeutic relationship.

Deep issues can arise, and it can seem as though the client's process is being cut across when an ending is effectively forced on them. While there will be instances where time may be available for a client to overrun, often the overrun will be into the time that the counsellor needs between clients. What is best is for clients to be gently reminded during the session how much time is left as the end time is approached. This may enable the client's internal process to adjust to the time available. Of course, there may be times when the client is actually deeply involved in an experience emerging from depth, so that the reminder does not impact on their awareness. In such instances the counsellor needs to be mindful of their own time constraints and those that the client may be subject to – a bus to catch home, a lift, an appointment to make after the session. It should not be assumed just because the counsellor may have time to overrun that the client is in the same position.

Carrie sniffed. 'I hate . . .', she swallowed, 'I hate everything.'
Sally instinctively nodded, she was still holding Carrie's arm, she gave it another gentle squeeze as she responded, 'so much to hate.
Carrie nodded. 'I hate being at home, I hate being at school, I hate being . . . , being . . . , me.' The tears became more copious and her sobbing more intense.
'So much to hate – home, school and you hate being you.'
'I-I wish everything was different. I get really sad, you know?'
'Yeah, all of it,' Sally nodded, 'leaves you so sad.'
'Sometimes it's OK, but sometimes I feel, you know, just really depressed.' She took a deep breath, the sadness was very present.
Sally responded, wanting to maintain her empathic appreciation of what Carrie was describing about how she felt. 'Hmm, that's a hard place to be, depressed.'
'Everything feels so dark, so hopeless.' Carrie wasn't so much thinking about what she was saying, she was just expressing, describing, what it was like, how she felt. It was so close, so present, so much how she could be. She sniffed and swallowed, reaching for another tissue and blowing her nose. 'Oh God,' she blew again, 'I-I drink sometimes to try and feel better.'

Sally nodded, feeling a flood of warmth for Carrie as she made her disclosure. She knew that it couldn't have been an easy thing to say, but perhaps it had emerged out of the desperation for help that was probably present within Carrie.

'I'm sure you do, and it helps, does it?'

'Sometimes, not always. Sometimes it makes it worse.'

'Drinking makes the feeling depressed worse?' Sally voiced her empathic response with a questioning tone, inviting Carrie to elaborate if she wished.

'Can do. It's best when I just, you know, pass out. I can get away from everything. I like that.'

'That feeling of getting away from it, you like that.'

Carrie nodded. She knew she was aware of knowing how at times she wished she was dead, but she didn't say anything. She felt anxious as she thought about it, her heart was thumping. She sniffed again and reached for another tissue as she felt more tears spilling over her eyelids. 'I wish everything was different.'

'If only, if only it could all be different.'

Carrie could feel her depression more intensely, and her sadness, and despair, and so many feelings, but she wasn't sitting there attaching names to them. It was like one, huge, sad and suddenly very lonely feeling. She so wished everything could be different. She took a deep breath, it felt awful and, at the same time, felt good to feel that someone was with her, listening, taking her seriously. It felt like . . . , she wasn't sure what, but there was a sort of sense of . . . , yes, a kind of relief somehow. But she still felt sad, and anxious as she sat there, dabbing at her eyes with the tissue.

'Must look a mess!' She tried to smile, but it was a struggle.

Sally smiled. 'It's certainly rearranged your make-up.'

The note of humour felt good, somehow, and she did manage a smile. But she couldn't sustain it and her face became serious again. 'Why does it have to be like this?'

'Why does it have to be, what, everything?' Sally wasn't sure if there was anything specific Carrie was referring to, she didn't know exactly what she was thinking as she heard the words.

'Life. Having crap parents. Everyone always telling you what to do.'

Sally nodded. 'That "why?".'

Carrie nodded. 'Yes', she thought, 'that "why?".' 'Why don't people listen to me, like you do?'

Sally felt herself catch her breath, she felt deeply touched by what was being said, by the yearning to be listened to that she sensed was being communicated to her by Carrie.

'I guess not everyone knows how to listen.' Sally was careful as she didn't want to say that not everyone wanted to listen and give the impression that she thought that Carrie's parents didn't want to listen. The truth was she had no idea what was happening for Carrie's parents. Maybe they didn't know how to listen rather than not want to listen, full of their own problems and stresses, perhaps. Though as she thought that she also felt that nevertheless parents really did need to listen to their children. But it seemed that something had stopped them from doing so, at least so far as Carrie was experiencing them.

'I just wish people would leave me alone.'

To Sally it felt as though what Carrie just said had really come from the heart. It was the way she had spoken. 'That's really heartfelt, so wanting to be left alone.'

Carrie sat, feeling sad, feeling tearful. She nodded, she was looking down. 'Do what I want.'

'Do the things that you want to do.'

'I hate it at home, it's always so tense. I hate it, I hate it so much.'

'Yeah,' Sally took a deep breath, 'yeah, you hate it so much.'

Carrie could feel herself tensing up as she spoke. She sat in silence again, feeling as though there wasn't really anything else to say. It all seemed so hopeless and she longed to get away, get on with her life. That's what she lived for, that and having a laugh, messing around with the boys and, yeah, drinking and feeling pissed. She loved that feeling of being 'out of it', that sort of spaced-out sensation in her head. That's where she wanted to be now, and just to sleep and fuck it all. Yeah, she thought, that's what she wanted, fuck it all. She took a deep breath and sighed.

'Big sigh.'

I don't like feeling depressed, but when I do, well, it's like I don't care. That's how it is.'

'Takes you to another place where you don't care.'

'Just feel so trapped.' Carrie thought about it and realised what she had said applied to how she felt when she was like that, but also how she felt at home. 'Yeah, trapped.'

'So trapped.' Sally spoke softly, it felt a very intense moment. She could hear a note of resignation in Carrie's voice, and it seemed to her, Sally, that Carrie just had so little energy left to fight it, to release herself, like she was slipping more deeply into the trap. 'Like you can't break free.'

Yes, Carrie thought, all feels too much, too heavy. Her thoughts were back to her parents. 'I wish they'd stop rowing. They get me depressed. I never, ever want to be like they are. I want to enjoy myself. Be a mum some day, yeah, have kids, but I'll be different, I know I will; I'll look after my kids. I know what it's like. They'll have what I didn't get, I'll be a good mum.' As she spoke there was a belief in what she was saying and a sense that Carrie was convincing herself that she was different as well.

'That sounds really strong and clear, you'll be a good mum, give your kids what you didn't get.'

Carrie felt a surge of emotion as words formed in her mind in response to what Sally had said. She'd felt herself about to say, 'I'll give them love', yet in the moment of thinking it she felt such a sense of not being loved, of not feeling loved, of feeling ignored, put down, moaned at, but the overwhelming feeling was of not feeling loved. She closed her eyes, it was a horrible, horrible feeling. She felt suddenly quite shaky, a strange tingling feeling, and her stomach felt like she was feeling sick. She swallowed. It stayed with her. Not feeling loved, and she could hear her parents' voices, shouting, always shouting, or silent, and she felt like she was invisible to them. Not to herself, she felt so full of so many awful feelings, but to them, it could feel like she wasn't there.

'Everyone shouts in our house.' She was shaking her head again. The emotions remained strong. She was afraid to say what she was really feeling. The words were stuck in her throat, but the feelings felt like they were screaming inside her body.

'Everyone shouts.'

'I just go to my room or I walk out. Sometimes I end up shouting as well, only way to get heard, 'cept you don't, not really.' She paused. She looked searchingly at Sally. 'You listen, don't you?'

'I try to.'

'It's important. Feels weird, yeah, but it's good as well.' She wasn't completely sure exactly why she was saying this, it was sort of a sense that she had.

Sally had noticed the time, and it was close to the session needing to end. 'I'm aware of the time. I don't want to cut across what you are experiencing, and we could take a few extra minutes if that would help, but I want to check how you are.'

'Tired. But it's sort of good. I mean, I've not really talked about, you know, like I have with you. It's not easy, Makes me feel upset, but that's not unusual. But, yeah, this is good, good to, yeah, you know?'

Sally nodded. 'Good to feel listened to, you mean, even though it's a bit weird?'

'Yeah, but . . . , yeah, it's OK.' She nodded, thinking about it but not really drawing any conclusion. 'Yeah.'

The session drew to a close. Sally conveyed again her sense that Carrie needed to look after herself as she left, that the session had been intense. Carrie agreed but said she was used to feeling like that. She'd be OK. She could handle it. She left feeling sad, and although the anxiety had faded, she did feel a bit low, and at the same time felt good about Sally. She didn't try to make sense of it, that was how it was. She felt sort of in a bit of a bubble. The world around her felt sort of distant. As she sat on the bus on the way home she was still very quiet. That was how, more than anything else, the session had left her feeling. Sort of quiet. She didn't want to go straight home. She decided to go down to the shopping mall, see who was around. She got out her mobile, thinking about who to call.

Sally sat back in her chair, feeling the intensity of the session. She felt she was beginning to connect so much more now with Carrie. Yes, still not much being said about the drinking, and, yes, she felt concerned for Carrie's mood, but then that was how Carrie had been for a while and she was finding her ways of coping. And now she at least had the counselling as well which, although it wasn't easy, was perhaps helping Carrie to move towards a contrasting relational experience to what she was used to. And, well, time would tell as to how that affected her, but she felt accepting that it would have a constructive effect. But she also knew that she wanted to address the actual drinking with Carrie, and while that was important, and she knew it was the real risk factor, it was a symptom, an effect, and she believed whole-heartedly that sustainable change required a person to address causes, not simply change the behaviours that resulted from them. She felt for Carrie, but she sensed a resilience in her as well. If she didn't feel that then she felt she would be more concerned. She took out her file and started to write her notes for the session.

Points for discussion

- How has the session left you feeling? What is most present for you, and why?
- How effective do you feel Sally has been in her responses to Carrie? How has she conveyed her unconditional positive regard for Carrie, and do you feel she has achieved this sufficiently?
- Were there any times in the session when you felt you would have responded differently? And, if so, what might you have said, and why?
- Do you feel the session reflected the principles of person-centred working? In what way?
- What would you take to supervision from this session?

Write counselling notes for this session as if you were Sally.

CHAPTER 9

Counselling session 3: information given that the client does not want to hear

Thursday 2 July

The session had begun. Carrie had said a little about her past week, how it had been for her, how she had felt 'sort of strange for a while', 'sort of quieter', 'not so sort of depressed', but 'really sort of wrapped up in my own thoughts', and then she'd met up with mates and she'd 'sort of forgotten about it, but hadn't as well'. It had returned again later. She'd just been aware of feeling quiet. Not quite so sad, somehow. She wasn't sure how else to describe it.

Sally had felt good about what Carrie was telling her. Sometimes she recognised it could be that a session could be quite intense, the client's emotions pulled this way and that, but then, once it all settled back down then something had changed. It was often hard to pinpoint exactly what had changed, maybe everything sort of tumbled back in a different sort of order. The image of a kaleidoscope was one that often came to her mind when she thought about this process. It was like, in the session, the kaleidoscope gets twisted slightly, and maybe not very much, and the pieces of glass start to tumble around. The client feels themselves in that sort of confused state in some way. And when they leave, or perhaps sometimes after, it's like the twisting has stopped and the pieces have settled into their new places, forming a new pattern. Same pieces, but a different arrangement. She didn't want to take the metaphor too literally, but it felt to her like it captured something of the process. And once the tumbling stops it's like it all goes quiet, and then there's a period of in some way getting to know what's new, what's different.

Carrie had stopped speaking. She felt she'd said everything about her week. Now she wasn't sure what to say. 'What do people talk about? I mean, I'm here because of my accident, but we don't talk about that.'

'Well, sometimes other things are more pressing. I want you to feel you can talk about what is most pressing and urgent for you. It's all linked, isn't it?'

Carrie nodded. 'So it's like, yeah, we haven't talked much about what happened, but, yeah, I suppose what we talk about is linked. I don't want to stop drinking, though.'

'Mhmm, I know.'

'But you don't tell me what to do, not really, you don't do you?' Carrie was frowning slightly.

'No, but I guess that's what you expected.' Sally paused, aware herself of how they hadn't really addressed Carrie's drinking, and that probably others might frown on the way she worked, that she should have addressed it straight away. But would Carrie have listened? Would she have just reacted against another adult who thought they knew best telling her what was good for her? It had been mentioned, but it had felt like it was something Carrie didn't want to hear. No, she was OK with the way she worked. She wanted to form the relationship and, without doubt, that was forming. The session had started very differently from the previous sessions, and there was more of a sense of communication and contact, maybe engagement was a better word.

'I suppose I've been thinking a bit about it this week. I sort of feel a bit sort of different about it.'

'About?' Sally wasn't sure exactly what Carrie was referring to.

'My drinking, wanting to get pissed. Feeling quiet made me sort of feel like I didn't want to get pissed, like I sort of didn't need to. That was weird.'

'Weird feeling like that, like you didn't want to get pissed.'

'Yeah. So, you know, it sort of made me think that I haven't said much about drinking and stuff. I haven't really, have I?'

'Not very much.' Sally thought about adding, 'is there something more you want to say?', but decided against it. She wasn't going to push Carrie, she wanted Carrie to feel a sense of her own autonomy in the relationship, feel her own power to choose, and for her own process to be free to express itself when it wanted to.

Carrie sort of wanted to say more and somehow this felt OK, like she felt she'd be taken seriously. That sort of made it feel easier, though it still felt strange. But she did want someone to understand her, someone who wouldn't keep interrupting her, telling her what to do, telling her she was wrong. She'd had that and didn't want that from anyone else. And yet, outside on the edge of her awareness, there was a small voice inside herself that so desperately did want someone who really cared, who really loved and understood her, to tell her what to do. But it was too quiet to feel heard, and too threatening to the sense of self that Carrie had constructed in response to how she had been related to over the years. It wasn't even strong enough to provoke anxiety, because it couldn't threaten to emerge sufficiently to impact on her awareness.

Mearns and Thorne (2000) have written about what they term 'edge of awareness' material, elements that are present within the organism's experience, but are not present in the person's awareness. If such experience is not congruent with the person's self-concept, and is being denied to awareness, it becomes lodged on the edge of the individual's awareness. As it threatens to emerge into awareness, then anxiety becomes the organism's response to this process.

'There isn't anything wrong in drinking, I mean, I'm not always drunk like mum. But, well, some days I just go for it, things get me down, want to, you know? Depends on what I'm feeling.'

'It sounds really important that you don't drink like your mum, and what you drink or how much sort of depends on how you are feeling.'

Carrie nodded. 'They told me I had to stop, you know, and they said it again when I had to go back last week for them to check on my arm. So I fell over, you know, but that doesn't mean I've got to stop drinking. If everyone who fell over had to stop drinking that'd be crazy. Told me I was harming myself and I just, well, I don't feel like it's harming me. All my mates drink, so what?' Carrie could feel herself becoming quite angry and irritated. She hated being told what to do, and she certainly hated the idea of not drinking. That was ridiculous as far as she was concerned, just justified her in thinking that she was being told things that were stupid.

'Sounds like it pisses you off, and the fact that all your mates drink means it's OK for you, that it's not harming you.'

Carrie pulled a face. 'Well, yeah.'

Sally nodded. She knew that what Carrie was saying was true for her in the sense that it was her perception, yet she was also aware that heavy alcohol use was damaging, that bingeing could put a person at risk – and more so a young person – and that it could cause health problems – and not just the effects of falling over – as well as other problems such as social, familial, financial, legal and, for young people of course, educational as well. As a person-centred counsellor she sought to remain within her client's frame of reference, but she knew that she had knowledge about alcohol and its effects, which it seemed clear that her client was not aware of. So, her client's perception, while it was her own and therefore true to what she knew, was in a sense partial and incomplete.

'Did the doctor or nurses give you any information about binge drinking?'

Carrie nodded, they had given her a leaflet, she hadn't read it, hadn't wanted to. Didn't like the idea they were suggesting she had a problem. Her mum did, but she didn't. Why didn't they talk to her mum? That was her thought about it all. No, she didn't have a problem, she looked away from Sally.

Sally noted the head movement. Carrie clearly didn't want to respond to her question. Sally felt she wanted to try and engage Carrie on the topic of the dangers of binge drinking. She felt that it hadn't been addressed, and now, well, now it seemed to be a topic that had become part of the therapy session.

> While it may be part of the therapy session, it is clearly a topic that the client is making clear she does not want to engage with. Therefore, continued emphasis on this is emerging more and more from the therapist's frame of reference and less and less from the client's. The non-directivity of the person-centred approach is being compromised. The client's belief about the relative safety of her own drinking is, from her perspective, being threatened. Unless or until her thoughts and feelings are such that she is open to a different perception, she will seek to defend her perception. This is what human beings do, particularly in relation to behaviours that are important to them, and even more so those with which the person has invested a sense of their own identity. The latter may not be the case here, except that Carrie sees herself as being a normal drinker, like her mates, like everyone else, and certainly not like her mum. This aspect of her identity, her self-concept, is being threatened. The counsellor needs to back off, and continue to work on offering empathy and unconditional positive regard. The relational experience, the offering of information must be in the context of empathy and unconditional positive regard, otherwise it will cut across the therapeutic relationship, and information will most likely be perceived or experienced as being given advice or, worse, being told what to do. In this instance this would feed straight into an aspect of Carrie that clearly does not want this. It would serve to undermine the therapeutic relationship further. Sally's response below leads to an exchange that is not always person-centred therapy. The counsellor has got lost in her own agenda. It is a supervision issue.

'You may have read it, maybe not, but bingeing puts your health at risk, and continued bingeing or heavy alcohol use can leave you with an alcohol habit that can be hard to break later.'

'But everyone drinks, I mean, you know, it's what everyone does. Why pick on me?'

'That's how it feels, that you're being picked on.'

Carrie nodded, feeling suddenly defiant. 'No one else gets told to stop.'

'Well, you did get drunk and break your arm, and the medical staff were no doubt concerned. And I can appreciate that it isn't what you want to hear, but alcohol is a danger to your health when it's not treated with respect.'

'But I feel good when I drink, mostly.'

'Yes, it has that effect, as you say, mostly.'

'I don't drink every day, not like mum does, and dad does sometimes.'

Sally thought momentarily how often parental drinking was seen as reason enough to drink by young people, parents not treating alcohol with respect, and then children following a similar path. Not always, she knew it wasn't a simple cause and effect relationship, but it was a contributing factor in her view to young people developing problems. 'Yes, your drinking isn't the same as theirs, and what I'm hearing you say is that because it isn't like the way they drink, then it's not a problem – because the way you drink is similar to the way that your mates do.'

Carrie nodded.

'I do hear you, Carrie, it simply doesn't feel like a problem to you.'

> The counsellor has brought the focus back on her client's experience and perception, where it should have been anyway.

Carrie shrugged. 'So I was sick, it happens, I fell over, yeah, so?'

Sally nodded and felt again that Carrie was not appreciating the seriousness of what had happened in terms of the risks to herself. She felt clearly that her respect for her clients demanded of her that if she had special knowledge in relation to alcohol use and its effect, that she should offer this to her clients.

> As highlighted before, where a person-centred counsellor feels that there is information to be offered to a client, then it must be offered in an atmosphere of unconditional positive regard for the client, out of a sense of warmth for the client, and with an empathic sensitivity to the client's perception. It must also not be given with an attitude of 'I know best', but offered perhaps gently, tentatively. The 'I know best' style is likely to provoke a reaction, a resistance, for the reasons mentioned previously. The client will defend her sense of self, the therapeutic relationship may be damaged, the endeavour to equalise the power relationship in the therapy room will be undermined.
>
> Having said this, some clients will make it clear that they do want to understand their drinking more, do want advice and information and some ideas for what they should do. The person-centred counsellor must be responsive to the client's frame of reference, to their expressed needs. And if the client genuinely wants information that the counsellor does not have, the counsellor should refer them on to someone who does.

Sally sensed that she had been too pushy in the way she had been speaking. She realised that she needed to offer what she knew more sensitively. It wasn't what she said that would encourage a client to hear, but the way it was said which, in turn, needed to be expressive of her warmth for her client, her unconditional positive regard. She spoke more softly, not deliberately so, but because that was how she felt she wanted to be. What she knew was likely to be difficult to hear. She hoped their relationship was strong enough to bear it.

'I know it probably doesn't sound serious, being sick, but people do die when they're sick when they've been drinking. Anyone who passes out from drinking too much, or falls asleep whilst under the influence of alcohol can, well, in effect drown in their vomit. Alcohol affects the breathing reflex, and heavy drinking is not good news. And I know it's not something widely known, but it is true. And I want you to be aware of it. I want you to make your own choices, Carrie, but there are things about alcohol that people need to know so that their choices can be informed and safe.' She kept her attention on Carrie as she spoke. As she finished, Carrie had turned to look at her once again. She nodded slightly as she caught Carrie's eyes. Sally felt a surge of warmth and caring for Carrie. Yes, she hoped she would listen, take it seriously. And she guessed how difficult that was likely to be for her. She hoped what she had said, and the way she had said it, would be heard and even if it didn't cause a change in behaviour, maybe it might sow a seed for another time. She felt she was being thoroughly authentic both in what she was saying and how she was feeling as she was speaking.

Carrie had listened to what Sally was saying. She had felt a reaction as Sally had been speaking. She didn't like being told what to do, and yet . . . Somehow she felt a little different. The room felt quiet. Sally sort of seemed to care, really care, she could see it in her eyes. Somehow she now didn't feel the same as when her parents or teachers told her what to do. This was different, and she was unsure. It was different, a little uncomfortable. She wasn't sure what to say. And she was also aware that when Sally had begun speaking a part of her had felt 'good, sometimes I want to die', but she also knew that she didn't, not really. It all felt too confusing.

'But why do I have to stop?'

'Why do you have to stop – that's what seems so unfair, yes?'

'I don't want to stop.'

'Mhmm.'

'But they said I had to.'

Sally was aware that in herself she felt strongly that it wasn't about stopping, it was about treating alcohol with respect, being aware of the dangers, the risks; being aware of why alcohol was important in a person's life. Yet she also didn't want to contradict what the medical staff had been saying either, leaving Carrie with mixed responses. 'I guess they were concerned. You had done yourself damage.'

'I suppose so. Doesn't seem fair though.'

'Yeah, doesn't seem fair. And what I'm hearing is, Carrie, and maybe I'm wrong, but that having a drink is important to you. It gives you something that you like, something that you don't want to lose. And what's being said is that your choice comes with a risk, particularly binge drinking, and you've already experienced aspects of that risk. Does that make sense?' Sally felt wholly genuine in what she was saying. It came from the heart. She wanted to empathise with both the spoken and the unspoken. She thought that maybe what she had said might offer Carrie the opportunity to choose whether or not to agree with her, that it might make things a little clearer.

'I suppose it does.' She sat and thought for a moment, tightening her lips as she did so. 'But it makes me feel good. Life's crap, I need to feel good.'

Sally nodded instinctively and felt herself taking a deep breath. What Carrie had said, and how she had said it, the feelings behind her words, made an impression and touched her deeply. 'What can I say, yeah, your life feels crap and alcohol brings you relief, a way to feel good.'

'A way to escape.'

'Yes, a way to escape as well.'

'But what you're saying is that I have to find other ways to feel good.'

'I guess I am. I mean, I don't want to say you have to, but to say that, well, given the risks, it's something to seriously think about.'

'Hmm.' Carrie lapsed into silence, trying to imagine what it would be like if she didn't drink, or drank less. The idea of drinking less had come into her mind. But that would mean no more oblivion, and she wanted that, needed that. She didn't like it. She looked across at Sally. Did she understand? Did she, really? She couldn't know what it was like, the rows, the angry silences that could seem as bad as the rows, worse sometimes, feeling so cut off, not really wanting to go home sometimes, hating so much, just wanting to get away from it all, get a life of her own, feel good, have fun, have a laugh and, yeah, when she wanted to, get pissed as well. What could she know about any of that?

The question stayed with her. As she looked at Sally she tried to make sense of her. Who was she? Did she really want to listen to her, or was it just a job to her? And yet ... She thought back, it had felt good talking earlier, she had felt listened to. But ... she wasn't sure. She wanted to live her own life, make her own choices, yeah, make her own choices. Sally's words were back in her head, 'I want you to make your own choices'. Well, yeah, so did she, but Sally seemed to be saying she was making crap choices.

The problem with expressing a view from one's own frame of reference as the counsellor is that you have no idea what meaning the client will attach to it from theirs. The counsellor had been seeking to extend the client's awareness, and to convey how she respects the client's right to make her own choices. But the client hears it as telling her that her choices are crap. She could be at risk of now judging herself in the context of the, to her, external locus of evaluation of the counsellor. If the client's internal locus of evaluation is weak and easily undermined, she may now take the view that not only are her drinking choices crap, but she might internalise this and extend it to all her choices. This would be far from therapeutically helpful, indeed, it would be extremely damaging, potentially leaving the client with a self-concept of being a person who makes crap choices.

What is said by the counsellor should not encourage the client to make different choices simply because of what the counsellor has told them. This is why the power relationship in therapy is crucially important, and why it is emphasised so strongly in the person-centred approach. Where there is strong imbalance, where a client feels they have to see things or behave in a particular way because of what a counsellor says, then it is undermining the client's ability to strengthen their own internal locus of evaluation and actually adding to the presence of 'conditions of worth'. Clients should be feeling encouraged to trust their own inner promptings, and for their choices to be the result of freely weighing up new information with what they already think and feel.

Carrie had looked up at the clock and noted that the session was soon due to end. She was glad. She felt like she'd had enough. She wanted ... , well, no, she didn't want to go home, but she did want to go.

Sally was also aware of the time, she'd noticed Carrie's glance at the clock. She also felt it was important to respond to Carrie's silence. 'You looked deep in thought, Carrie, I didn't want to interrupt. But our time is nearly up today. My fantasy is that it wasn't easy hearing some of the things I said about risks associated with binge drinking. I want you to know what you are doing, Carrie, I see you as someone with a lifetime ahead of you, and I accept that you need to make the choices that feel right for you, now.' Sally felt she was expressing genuinely held thoughts and feelings. She spoke with an air of authority, not an authority over anyone, but it was an air that was expressive of the genuineness and authenticity in what she was saying.

Carrie listened. The way Sally spoke did seem to be for real, like she wasn't just sort of saying it for effect. She wasn't used to that. She didn't quite know what to make of it. She suddenly felt sad, tearful, it felt like someone cared. But she also knew as well that she didn't want to do something because someone told her to do it. Yes, she did want to make her own choices, live her own life. But she didn't want to mess up. She sighed. She didn't know. She really didn't know.

'I don't know what to do. I guess I need some time to think, a bit of space, you know? I don't know. I don't want to be depressed, hate that. I want a laugh, mess around, feel good.' She thought of the clothes she liked to wear. Yeah, that made her feel ... , yeah, that was it, made her feel. Not always feel good, just made her sort of feel, yeah, like she was someone.

'Have a good time, yes?'

Carrie nodded. 'Yeah.' She paused. 'Got to go.'

They discussed a next appointment – Carrie agreed to come back the next week. She headed off for the bus home. She wanted, yeah, to feel good but sometimes she just wanted to feel like she was herself somehow. Sort of strange that. She hated being at school, and being who she was sometimes. Who was she? The question stayed with her as she walked along the path to the bus stop. She didn't want to be her mother's daughter, and she certainly didn't want to think of herself as a schoolgirl, yeeeagghh, hated that. She wanted to be herself, express herself. She liked dark colours and dark make-up. Made her feel like she was someone. That felt right, OK, good. She continued to walk towards the bus stop.

Sally, meanwhile, was left feeling very uncertain and quite troubled. It had not felt an easy session. Was easy the right word? No, she didn't feel it had gone well, felt she'd said too much, lost her empathy. But she wanted Carrie to have information. It was difficult. She knew she needed to take the session to supervision. It was difficult, she knew as a counsellor within a specialist setting, and with a specialist remit – was she strictly therapeutically focused or was it OK to share information? And was it either or? Could it be both? Why not? But then, she believed the therapeutic relationship was the key factor and, yes, she knew that it was that which sort of created the context within which information could be offered. And she knew that many young people did want information and advice, but not always to be left with a sense that they were being told what to do. It was getting the balance right, getting alongside the young person. It wasn't always easy.

She felt it right to not hold back information that was relevant to what the client brought to the counselling sessions, or where it was health related. She was, after all, working within a healthcare system at the hospital. She wondered if she would be different in a different setting if Carrie was her client. She thought probably not. It wasn't the setting, it was her as a human being, a human reaction – maybe a motherly reaction? Yes, she did want Carrie to have what she needed to make healthy choices, and she could well appreciate that Carrie believed she was making healthy choices because they helped her feel better.

Points for discussion

- What thoughts and feelings are you left with having read this session?
- How do you feel about giving information to clients? How do you feel it should be done in order to preserve the therapeutic relationship? Or should it not be done at all?
- How might you have responded during the session to what Carrie was saying, or how she was being?
- Do you feel that Sally managed to restore her empathic responding to Carrie after losing touch with the client's frame of reference? What are the theoretical implications of the counsellor shifting into her own frame of reference?
- Consider the notion that constructive personality change involves a client moving from an external to an internal locus of evaluation. What is it that the person-centred counsellor offers to encourage this?
- What specific issues would you take to supervision from this session?

Write counselling notes for this session.

CHAPTER 10

Supervision session: restoring counsellor congruence

Tuesday 7 July

'I don't think I handled the last session with my new client at all well.' Sally sat
not feeling too pleased with herself and just generally feeling that she needed
time to explore what had happened with her supervisor, Ros. They had
worked together for a couple of years now and both were used to each other's
style of working. Sally began to describe to Ros the background to Carrie
attending for counselling and what had been the context of the sessions so
far. Ros listened attentively, committed to offering her supervisee the same
therapeutic conditions that she offered her clients, seeking to encourage an
open, facilitative environment in which her supervisees would feel free to
explore themselves, their clients and their reactions to their clients. She
wanted supervisees to feel supported and able to bring their process into the
supervision session.

For Ros, supervision was a collaborative process, co-professionals exploring the
relational, therapeutic process, checking out the quality of the supervisees'
empathic responding, acknowledging and encouraging the presence of warm
acceptance of the client and exploring where it was felt that it was not present,
and ensuring that the supervisee could maintain a congruent presence and feel
a sense of being integrated into the therapeutic relationship, in contact with
the client.

'OK, so, that gives me some background and a sense of your client. Clearly Carrie
has a lot happening for her, a lot to cope with and she's coping, at least in part,
with alcohol, we don't know to what degree and we don't know what else she
might be using or doing to cope with what she is experiencing. Her mood is
fluctuating, she goes silent and feels to you as if she goes quite distant and
detached, leaving you feeling concerned or uncertain about the degree of contact between you.'

Two points worth considering. First of all, the supervisee names the client in supervision. Some supervisees will do this, others not. Personally, I find that the bringing of the client's name into the supervision session helps to personalise the person being described. The risk is that the supervisor may associate the name with someone else, and that might obstruct hearing what the supervisee is saying. Counsellors and supervisors must make their own minds up on this.

Secondly, the issue of not feeling in contact. How little contact is needed for contact to be enough? So long as the client is aware of the counsellor's presence, then one can argue that the relationship exists. Then comes the question as to whether the relationship can be defined as therapeutic. How much of the empathy and unconditional positive regard must the client be aware of, and how much of the counsellor's authenticity do they need to register, in order for the relationship to be described as therapeutic? It is not for the counsellor to judge. It is a matter for the client, with the counsellor seeking to consistently offer the therapeutic attitudes. The counsellor may doubt the contact if, for instance, the client seems unaware of their presence, perhaps if a psychotic episode occurs or perhaps during intense intoxication, although from my own experience I have known clients remember sessions when I felt that there was little contact, and have been surprised by what has been recalled.

Sally nodded. 'I mean, it would be easy to think of her mood shifts as being, well, a symptom of being a teenager, you know? Many do think that way, of course, and I believe that sometimes more serious problems can be missed because of this. However, that's another discussion. For me it is too simplistic. It's dismissive and it doesn't acknowledge the individuality of the client, of the young person themselves and that, for them, whatever is occurring for them, around them, within them, is a deeply personal and individual experience. It's their experience that needs to be heard and attended to, and validated and understood. So it might sound similar to other people, but it is still uniquely theirs. But you hear it, don't you, "oh, so and so is just being a teenager", "just another adolescent reaction, it'll pass". We're so good at that in our society, making sweeping generalisations. What good are they to the young person? Yes, OK, the behaviour, the attitude may be similar to others, but what is that individual young person actually experiencing? What is their story? What does it mean to them? What are their reasons for being the way they need to be?'

Ros was very aware of how Sally was speaking and she responded to this. 'You sound very passionate in what you are saying, Sally. It's really important to you, isn't it?'

'Yes, been there, I know what it's like and it's frustrating, very frustrating, and it provokes you, or at least that was how it affected me, to react more strongly.

But, well, maybe a bit of my past gets out sometimes, and, well, I am aware of it. So, yes, it is important to me. It does make me angry.'

'That's being general, and personal to you. Does Carrie's situation make you angry then?'

Sally thought for a moment. 'Yes, I guess it does. I haven't really felt that in the session, though, more a sense of sadness for her and yes, a real sense of compassion too. Here she is, 15 years old, parents rowing, mother drinking – well, they both seem to drinking though maybe with different patterns or styles. She hates home, sees them as "crap parents", her words, she hates school, hates herself, and just wants to get away.'

Ros again noted the passion in Sally's voice. 'She really draws feelings out of you, and she should be given the intensity of her experience. Fifteen years old and, well, surrounded by so much that she hates.'

'She does draw the feelings out of me, and thank God she does, you know? I want, need to be affected by my clients. What use am I to them if I am not? I remember reading some years ago in a book, and I can't find the quote now though it has stuck with me: "how can they feel our love if we cannot feel their pain?". That speaks to me, Ros, it really does.'

Ros felt herself taking a deep breath at Sally's words. 'Yes, yes, that really does convey something so powerful and, yes, so true. I like that, thanks for sharing it. Hmm. And Carrie brings a lot of pain?'

'She draws attention to it, well, I suppose she doesn't, I mean she doesn't talk specifically about pain, more about what she hates, but it must pain her for her to hate it.'

'Yes, so it's like the pain is present but not voiced.'

'But I see it in her face, when she is silent. She does not look at all comfortable.'

'You feel it?'

'I sense its presence, I see a 15-year-old girl trying to find a way through childhood, trying to cope with so many feelings, and I only know such a small part of her life and her experience. I don't know what has happened in the past, how her parents have been throughout her life, and what effect that will have been having. All I know is what I witness now, in the counselling room, a very sad young girl, hating so much and drinking to feel better. And that makes me sad and, yes, you're right, that also make me angry. Yes, it's that which makes me angry.' Sally was shaking her head.

The supervision has brought the counsellor's anger to the surface. It may or may not have been present in the session, it wasn't being directly experienced within the counsellor's awareness, but it has now emerged and can be acknowledged. The fact that it may have been present but not in the counsellor's awareness could have contributed to the counsellor's responses not being as empathic, accepting and non-directive as they might have been. By becoming aware of these feelings, and therefore more fully integrating them within her awareness, the counsellor will be more congruent and therefore offer a more effective therapeutic presence to the client.

'What's happened to her specifically?'

'That she has been put in this position.'

'That she's been put in the position of . . . ?'

'Having to feel what she is feeling and having to binge drink to deal with it, and find that drinking alcohol has become a major way for her to feel good. That is not good learning, and good preparation for adulthood.'

Ros nodded. Again, Sally was, well, the phrase that came to mind was, on a roll. Again that passion. 'That's what gets to you.'

Sally nodded. 'And you know, the sessions, they're really intense, it feels intense, the listening, the staying focused on Carrie during her silences. I don't really think about it like this at the time, you don't, you get absorbed into the process, can't think of a better way of putting it.'

'You feel absorbed into the counselling process?'

'Yes, and I want to say not "absorbed by" but "absorbed into", somehow that feels important.'

'Something important about being "absorbed into", that seems to mean something quite meaningful and specific.'

Sally nodded. 'It's like becoming the process, being the process, being in process, I'm not sure what other words to use. But, yes, I know what it is, it's like being less of an observer and more of a participant. Yes, that's the best way to put it.'

'Mhmm, so the process draws you in and you become more of a participant, at least you feel yourself as participating rather than observing.'

'Yes, hmm, but then, hmm, yes, when the detaching and distancing, yes, yes, that's when I begin to feel more of an observer. Now that's interesting, I hadn't thought of it like that before.'

'So, that sounds like the degree of contact somehow governs where you feel yourself to be on a sort of observer–participant continuum?'

Sally was nodding. She liked that. It made perfect sense. 'And I need to address what happens in order to cause me to lose that participative sense and feel like an observer who in a sense is one step back from what is happening for my client.'

'Right.'

In quantum physics it is recognised that in some mysterious way the observer is in fact a participant, that the act of observation can affect the outcome. Measuring light, for instance, depending upon whether you wish to measure its direction and movement or whether you wish to measure its position, will affect whether it appears to take the form of a wave or a particle. So, the act of observation becomes an act of participation.

However, two people in a counselling room are not engaging in a manner reflective of quantum physics, although the nature of the mind and the working of consciousness are not fully understood, and many suggest that both are phenomena that have a reality beyond the working of the physical brain. There is something, however, about the notion of counselling as a participative process, and perhaps particularly so in person-centred working, where there is no attempt to be detached from the client's process, where there is no attempt to analyse from psychological distance. Therefore the sense of participation is important and perhaps might be regarded as an indicator of therapeutic or, at least, relational contact. But where that experiencing tends towards observation, then there will have been a move away from the kind of relational contact that is one of the necessary conditions for therapeutic change within the person-centred system.

'And I'm thinking back to the sessions but also thinking about me, now, here, and how I am talking about them. Yes, you're right, there is passion there. I don't sort of think that way during the session, but then there isn't the reflective space in the way that there is here, now. And thinking about it, what I said earlier, feeling that I hadn't been too good in the last session, there is also something that maybe I'm on a bit of a mission here.'

'Can you say more?'

'Maybe I'm caring so much that I want to push Carrie along, you know? I'm thinking of how I raised the risks associated with her alcohol use. She doesn't like being told what to do, by anyone, she's told me that. And it wasn't that I exactly told her what to do, I sought to highlight the risks of binge drinking, but she heard it as criticism of her choices and as being told she had to do something else – not drink. And I tried to explain that I simply wanted her to make her own choices but that I wanted her choices to be informed.'

'Mhmm, so your sense now is that you may have been pushing her along and though you feel you weren't tending to tell her what to do, that was what she experienced.'

Sally nodded, and as she heard Ros's response she felt an uneasiness within herself. This was a distinct contrast to the passion she was feeling when she had been speaking earlier. Something wasn't right. She knew that feeling and it generally indicated that she wasn't being true in some way. 'I'm uneasy, Ros. What I'm saying, no,' she shook her head, 'no, there's something not right here. I can't just, well, sound like I'm blaming the client for how she heard me; maybe my words were to raise her awareness around binge drinking but my purpose was more than that. I don't want her to mess up her life ...' Sally went silent, recalling something that she had said during the session. 'Hmm.'

'Hmm?' Ros raised her eyebrows as she responded, inviting more from Sally.

'I'd also said something, at least I think I did, I'm sure I did, and if I didn't well I certainly thought it, but I think I said something like, 'you have your whole life ahead of you'. She shook her head. 'What a stupid thing to say, and how patronising was that? Of course she has her whole life ahead of her. Talk about stating the obvious, as if Carrie isn't aware of that although, well, I do know as well that young people can sometimes live with an attitude of not looking too far ahead.'

'Generalisation.'

'I know.' Sally felt herself taking another deep breath, and sighed, 'yes, I know.' She paused before moving on to another topic. 'It's that tension between being purely therapeutic as a person-centred counsellor, and having information that the client probably isn't aware of and which could help them make more healthy choices. But then, well, in a way she is making what feels to her like a healthy choice, binge drinking – it makes her feel better, different, brings relief. But it isn't healthy, and while it brings temporary relief, it isn't lasting, it isn't a long-term solution, just dampens down the feelings a bit, sometimes at least. She also talked about how alcohol lowers her mood when her mood is already low. I think she does get down, I mean she used the word "depressed" herself. I don't know how deep, but it is clearly a reaction to her circumstances – I'm tempted to say quite a healthy reaction in a way, quite realistic – and then the alcohol is another unwelcome factor, however much it feels like it helps.'

Depression is a symptom, an effect. One of the problems with mental health services in general is that they are geared up to treat symptoms and not causes. This is different from physical medicine. Someone has a stomach pain, the doctor does not treat the stomach pain but seeks to ascertain the cause and treat that. It could be an ulcer and therefore action is taken to try and heal it. But it may be a problem requiring surgery. Physical medicine seeks out the underlying cause and treats that, as well as giving symptom relief where that is necessary. Any diagnosis will not be 'stomach pain' but 'ulceration' or 'inflamed gall bladder', the cause, not the effect.

With mental health the usual diagnoses such as depression, anxiety, panic attacks, personality disorder, schizophrenia, bipolar disorder and the various behavioural syndromes that seem to have proliferated in recent years are effects, symptoms. In some cases, yes, they may well be the result of chemical imbalance requiring a chemical solution, but very often they are symptoms of experiential factors, of events that have had a damaging or a profoundly traumatic impact on the psychological functioning of the person. The need is to look beyond the symptoms and treat the cause. The difficulty with mental illness is that symptom relief can leave the person not feeling they need treatment, or they are affected by medication in such a way that the psychological and emotional processes are affected, perhaps to the detriment at times of the therapeutic process.

So, for instance, a young person with an anxiety disorder who is also depressed may actually be experiencing the psychological and emotional effects of sexual abuse. That is the cause and it can be argued that if there is to be a diagnosis then it should be that, 'target of sexual abuse'. Or in the case of Carrie, she has an alcohol problem developing, but actually the cause might be described as 'a lack of consistent love and parenting in child-hood'. That's the cause, and that should therefore be the diagnosis and the focus for treatment responses. A mental health system that operated in this way would be very different, treating causes as the primary response and symptom diagnosis and management as secondary.

'It seems like that is your difficulty, knowing what you know, and knowing, or at least assuming, that what you know is what she doesn't know.'

'I don't think that Carrie appreciates the risk of vomiting after drinking, the risk of asphyxiation. And I haven't said anything about the risk of actual alcohol poisoning and what happens when an alcohol habit gets ingrained. There just seems so much happening for her.'

'So much happening for her and, what my sense is, so much happening for you as well.'

'Only three sessions, a lot of silences, but yes, you're right, a lot going on for me. She has made an impression on me, an impact, a very human impact. And I need to be truly in touch with my reactions – clarify my congruence, as it were – so I can be clearer in myself when I am with her, and more fully aware of my reactions and what in me governs the nature of my responses to her.'

Ros nodded, hearing what Sally was saying and wondering quite how Sally would approach that. 'Mhmm, so, how do you want to approach that?'

'I feel like I am. Feels like I already have a clearer sense of myself and of the, yes, amount I care, and how ... , and there's something for me that's important about caring. I have to care, how effective am I if I don't?'

'It's important to care and to feel that care about our clients.'

'But it's the "I know best", or the "I know what you need to know", but I do know things!'

'Then maybe it becomes more a matter of when you share what you know and how you share it, and what is the focus within yourself that urges that sharing.'

'For me, it's about how do I share information with a client in a way that is therapeutically helpful, and with a client who, as with Carrie, is conditioned to expect to be told what to do, and who instinctively reacts against it.' Sally paused. Something she had said a little while back had come back into her thoughts. 'You know, here I am and what did I say a little while ago, about not thinking that Carrie understands what happens when an alcohol habit becomes ingrained? OK, so she may not appreciate the range of health complications, but she sees the psychological and relational damage every day – her mother. That must be ... ' Sally took a deep breath. 'I'm so full of my own thoughts and feelings that I wonder if I'm really empathising with hers. She's got to hear me, feel me appreciating, understanding her world. And there's a difference, as you know.'

Ros nodded.

In reality what is often experienced by a counsellor is empathic appreciation rather than empathic understanding. To truly understand means to have another's experience, and the counsellor does not have that. What they have is an empathic appreciation of what has happened to their client and how their client has been affected. They have an appreciation of the feelings, the thoughts, the behaviours that are present for the client and which the client seeks to communicate. It can be helpful to hold this distinction in mind. Not everyone will see it this way, but it feels important to make this

> differentiation, otherwise the counsellor can begin to think they understand their client and is at risk of saying that they understand. But they don't. The uniqueness of the client's experiencing is their own. At the same time, we might set aside the use of language and acknowledge that what is most important is that the counsellor's experiencing and awareness are touched by what is present for the client, and what the client communicates. That is what matters, whether you call it appreciation or understanding.

Sally was feeling uneasy again as a discomforting thought struck her. 'Am I avoiding going into Carrie's dark place with her?' She looked at Ros. Something in those last few words left her feeling uneasy and yet, at the same time, there was something that felt instinctively – or maybe it was intuitively – right about what she had said.

'A difficulty going to her dark places with her?'

'She's only 15.'

'Her age makes you feel different?'

Sally nodded. 'Not sure I feel . . . , oh dear, me feeling she needs an adult.'

'Maybe she does.'

'Hmm, maybe, but her conditioned sense of self doesn't want to hear an adult telling her what to do.'

'No, but that doesn't mean she doesn't also long for someone to tell her what to do, given what she is coping with.' Ros was aware that her response was more explorative than empathic, but she accepted that supervision opened that up within the supervisory dialogue.

'Like she has both feelings, both needs.' Sally took a moment to reflect on what was being suggested, and found herself nodding in agreement. 'That makes sense. But she's not showing me the part that may want answers as to what she needs to do. After all, she has found her way of coping.'

'Mhmm.'

'Hmm.' Sally looked towards the window. She needed a moment or two to collect her thoughts. Ros remained silent, recognising that Sally needed thinking space, time to be with what was present for her without external disruption.

'And it's an assumption that part of her wants answers from someone else.' Sally felt she wanted to be clear on that. She didn't want to become too focused on assumptions. They could be wrong, however reasonable they might appear, and they could lead counsellors into being a step ahead of their clients and being less sensitive to what the client was experiencing and communicating, or more concerned with whether what was being communicated fitted their assumptions.

'Yes.'

'But it's likely to be there.' Sally paused again. 'It's about trust, isn't it; it's about whether I can trust Carrie – maybe it's more than that, maybe it's doubt whether I can trust young people who are binge drinking.'

'You question whether you can trust young people who binge drink?' Ros responded questioningly, inviting further exploration, aware that what Sally had said seemed to have emerged quite suddenly, and perhaps now needed to be engaged with to be fully appreciated.

'There is an "I know best" in me. And it's getting in the way of me offering the therapeutic conditions. But I don't know what's actually best for Carrie. I know what is damaging and risky about the choices she is making now, but what is best for her, what is the way forward that she needs to take, that I do not know. And, well, the question it leaves me with is "can I trust her to find it?".' Sally nodded as she finished speaking, confirming to herself that she agreed with the statement she had made about herself.

'Mhmm, can you trust, really trust, Carrie to find her way forward?'

'And yet that's daft as well because she has found a way, she's living her way, what works best for her. It's me, I want to think that I know that there's a better way.'

'And you may be right, that in terms of risk and damage there may be a better way, but having that perception so present in your awareness . . .'

'. . . is what is disrupting my empathy. Hmm. I don't think it's upsetting my unconditional positive regard. I don't feel that my positive regard is conditional on her acting in a particular way. But, I am not conveying warm acceptance of her, am I? And I guess that means that my unconditional positive regard is compromised, it isn't as pure or clear . . .' Sally paused, '. . . or as authentic, maybe that's a better word, not as authentic as it needs to be. And how can Carrie develop feelings of genuine positive self-regard and of her own authenticity if I am not bringing the therapeutic conditions into the relationship?'

Another pause. Again Ros left Sally with her thoughts, and the thought struck Ros as she sat and maintained her presence was that she was in fact offering Sally the very thing that in a sense Sally had struggled, or was struggling, to offer Carrie – trust in her own process.

'So it's me. So easy to think it's the client, isn't it, blocking the process, making it untrustworthy but it's me.'

'Mhmm, you feel that it is you and I want to share a thought that I just had which was that, in effect, by my giving you the space to think here, now, I am demonstrating my trust in your process.'

Sally smiled. She caught on. 'Yes, yes, I know, and I can feel a reaction in me as well, I can immediately feel myself wanting to say "yes, but Carrie is only 15".'

'So we are back to the difficulty that you seem to be experiencing in trusting the client's process, trusting the presence of the therapeutic conditions in encouraging constructive personality change when you have a young client that is binge drinking.'

'And in that place, yes, I am right to not trust the therapeutic process because I am not offering the therapeutic conditions. OK, I have to back off, I have to hear what Carrie's life is like, really like, and not want to get in there with my "I know best", which I don't, and I have to convey that caring and warm acceptance of her as a young person, her as a person.' Sally paused as further thoughts came into her awareness. 'And, yes, it's not just conveying, there's something about keeping clear, keeping it clean, yes, being sure that my warm acceptance and caring is clean, pure, if you like, not tainted by an agenda, or an intention.'

'Can you say more?' Ros felt that what Sally was saying could be usefully explored a little further. Her response was an invitation.

'It's like what is my motive here? I have to be clear that my warm acceptance is offered simply as warm acceptance and not with an intention to make something happen – the "if I give you unconditional positive regard you'll show me unconditional positive self-regard". Yes, we know it happens, but let it happen, my focus is on what I feel and convey, and, yes, clear and clean are two words that seem particularly apposite here.'

'Clear and clean.' Ros nodded. They felt like good words, she liked them.

'And open, I have to be open. This is all helping me to get back to the essence of therapy which is about getting back to me with greater awareness. My concerns, my anxieties, yes, my distrust, they all take me away from Carrie. Hmm, well, no, what I maybe mean is that my not being fully aware of my own process – what it is in me that has influenced how I have been with Carrie – means that I haven't been congruent, have I? Not really.'

'Not congruent because these concerns, anxieties, in a sense their true basis was outside of your awareness. Is that what you mean?' Ros wanted to check that she was hearing Sally correctly and not misinterpreting her words. It felt important, particularly because there were subtleties involved and the insight was an evolving one within the session, and Sally did not need some unhelpful comment from her to distort the process.

'Yes, they were present in my experiencing, and were being communicated in what I was saying and how I was saying it, but I wasn't fully aware of what was happening. There wasn't a clear and open relationship in me between my experiencing, my awareness and my communication. I'd lost my congruence. But now it feels like this is restoring it. These elements were not in my awareness. And that's what I need, and what Carrie needs. And I can only hope that I haven't in some way damaged the therapeutic relationship or made it more difficult for Carrie to feel able to engage in the therapeutic process.'

Ros was nodding. 'Time will tell. She clearly reacted. And the next session, well, it will be interesting how this supervision session may have affected you.'

Sally smiled, but there was a seriousness behind the smile. 'I hope I am more openly available to her, for her. She doesn't need me telling her what she needs. I still know very little about her really, and maybe that's a symptom of her not trusting me enough to tell me, because of how I have been. I have to do better.'

'I think this has been a valuable piece of work. I know how seriously you take your work, there's a lot of learning in this.'

Sally agreed. The supervision session moved on to a consideration of other clients, and after the session Sally left feeling very much more open to herself as she thought about Carrie once more. Yes, she felt less unease, and was looking forward to endeavouring to be a more congruent therapist when they next met.

Points for discussion

- Were the issues addressed in the supervision that you felt needed to be addressed?
- Had you been Sally, would you have wanted more from Ros?
- Had you been Ros, would you have responded differently?
- How would you sum up the value of this supervision session in terms of person-centred theory and its role in helping prepare Sally for her next contact with Carrie?
- If you were Sally, what notes would you write to capture your insight and learning from this supervision session?

CHAPTER 11

Counselling session 4: an emotional release, the client feels 'lighter'

Thursday 9 July

Sally definitely felt a greater degree of clarity in herself as she waited for Carrie to arrive. She thought she'd been clear before, but obviously she hadn't been. She felt a renewed sense of wanting to listen to Carrie, to really listen to what she was thinking, feeling, experiencing. She felt relaxed, ready to accept her client. Yes, she could more easily and consciously accept openly to herself that she did feel she knew best, while also knowing that in reality she probably didn't. Yes, it was one thing to think Carrie needed to reduce or stop her drinking, but that didn't remove or change the cause of her drinking. Without alcohol, Carrie would still have to find coping mechanisms. If she didn't drink, what might she do instead if she still carried the feelings inside her that she used the alcohol to escape from or dampen down? Get no relief and so get more depressed? Feel suicidal with no relief, and maybe in desperation act on it – either as a call for help or to simply put a final end to it all? Start to cut herself, assuming she didn't do that already, though Sally felt that that might have been picked up on examination at A&E – though that assumed she cut on her arms, of course.

Sally's thoughts stayed with the risk of cutting. She was shaking her head as she thought about how people got to that point of being no longer able to bear emotional pain, and instead inducing physical pain as a way of relieving the pressure. It could feel like a pain they could manage, or a diversion, it could have so many different meanings. Like choosing to binge, each person cut for their reasons, and those reasons needed to be listened to and received with warm acceptance. Yes, she thought, Carrie has a coping mechanism. It's risky, but it's been working. What she needed now was therapeutic space to begin to feel able to reach behind the behaviour and perhaps allow what was inside her to be released. And for that to happen she needed to experience the therapeutic conditions. Sally had to be authentically present and warmly accepting of Carrie, and able to hear and appreciate what Carrie said, and Carrie had to be able to experience Sally's responses. And whatever happened within Carrie needed to happen at a pace that, well, that was in tune with the actualising tendency as it worked through her emotional and psychological processes.

It was a few minutes later and Carrie was in the counselling rooms. Sally recalled the end of the last session and wondered what Carrie would want to focus on. Sally felt a sense of assurance within herself as she opened up the dialogue.

'You left last time wanting time, space to think. I am wondering what you want to talk about today.'

Carrie had done some thinking after that last session and on and off during the week. She had felt a kind of inner conflict, at times feeling good about the counselling, about Sally and how she listened and cared. Yet at other times she had also wished she could just carry on the way she was and not have to think about things. Hearing Sally's voice again, she seemed ... , she wasn't sure. It left her feeling sort of chatty, somehow, something seemed more relaxed.

'I guess I'm sort of not sure about what to do. I mean, yeah, I sort of don't want to change but I do. It's been a crap week, again. Nothing ever changes. Mum drinking, dad getting angry, rowing, me keeping out of the way, going to my room, going out, meeting up with my mates, you know?'

'Mhmm, doing the usual things and another crap week.' Sally sought to sum it up quite briefly and allow Carrie to pick on whatever theme she wanted to develop further.

'Dad pisses me off. He's just, oh I don't know, he's so remote, like he's in his own world most of the time. He's obsessed with work. Seems to be what he spends all his time doing. He's got an office at home and he's always in there. I don't know what he does at work but he always seems to bring more home with him.' She shook her head. 'Always too busy. And he drinks as well when he's working, not like mum, but he does.' She took a deep breath. 'Never time for me.'

'So you feel, what, cut off from him?' Sally was thinking of the remoteness Carrie had referred to.

Carrie nodded. 'He just feels, oh I don't know, so awkward somehow, it's difficult to talk to him. I don't know, he's in his head all the time, so, so ... , oh I don't know, he's my dad, yeah, but he can feel so distant.'

'Hmm. So very distant.' Sally kept her response brief and focused, capturing what Carrie had finished by saying.

Often therapeutically effective empathy is not about repeating back what a client has said in total, or taking them back over the start of what they had just said. As a client speaks they are in process. The counsellor conveys their listening through their attention. By responding to the final thing that is said, the counsellor does not interrupt the flow, allowing the client to know they have been listened to and heard, but with the minimum of disturbance. The client is then able to continue. The continuation might be verbally, the client saying more, or it can be through silence as the client is held in the place they have reached, dwelling a little more deeply, or being more deeply in touch with what they have focused on.

Carrie lapsed into silence. She thought about home, took a deep breath and blew it back out with a sigh. 'Just feel so alone at home.'

'Home is a lonely place.'

Carrie nodded. 'If it wasn't for my friends, you know?'

Sally nodded. She spoke gently, it felt like an intense experience for Carrie. 'They're really important to you.'

'But when I get depressed, I don't want to see anyone.' Carrie paused. 'Strange, there were times when I've looked forward to coming here, it feels different. Sort of escape, sort of. But I don't like, you know, the things you said about alcohol, being told I have to stop drinking, you know? But, well, at least you listen, it feels different here.'

'Yeah.' Sally took a deep breath herself. 'Hearing about alcohol isn't nice, but something feels different about being here and there have been times when you've looked forward to it.' Sally was conscious of feeling relaxed and fully accepting of what Carrie had expressed. Yes, she could well imagine the mix of thoughts and feelings she must have been having. It sounded incredibly realistic. She had no reason to doubt it, and felt no urge to be defensive because, yes, she'd contributed to Carrie feeling she didn't want to come. She was glad, though, that Carrie had felt able to express both sides of her experience.

'You do still think I need to stop drinking, though?'

'I think you would put yourself at less risk if you drank less. But at the moment it helps, it's helping you cope with what you are feeling.' Sally spoke freely without hesitation. It was what she genuinely felt, and she also felt her warmth for Carrie as she spoke.

Carrie nodded. She didn't react. She didn't think about the fact that she hadn't reacted in the way that she had in the past. The reaction just wasn't there. 'Does make me feel like I'm sort of free of it all, for a while, then it's crap again.'

'Bit of a roller coaster – up and down?'

Carrie nodded again. She looked down – yes, up and down. She liked the up, hated the down. 'Sometimes I wish I could get off. I mean, you know, just get off.'

'Stop it all, no more ups and downs, just get off?'

'That's why I drink a lot sometimes. That's how I get off. I can forget it all then.'

Sally felt herself responding to this insight, it felt an important one that Carrie was owning for herself. She wanted to be sure that she had understood Carrie correctly so she sought to check it out in her response. 'So it's like there are ups and downs, but when you drink heavily that's like stepping off that roller coaster.'

'That's why I want to get away in the future, have my own space. Maybe I won't drink as much then.' Carrie paused. 'But then, I like the feelings it gives me. So maybe I'd just drink more.' Her mum came to her mind. 'But I mustn't be like mum.' She took a deep breath. It all felt too much.

Sally was about to respond, but Carrie added a little more. 'Yeah, I do like the feelings it gives me.'

Sally nodded and responded to what Carrie had just said. 'Those feelings are really important to you.' Sally felt a heartfelt warmth for Carrie as she listened to her and responded. She felt somehow more fluid in herself as she sat there, more able to go with the flow, less attached to an agenda.

Carrie felt sad, unsure, a bit confused, but at the same time it felt sort of OK to be talking, felt a little easier somehow. Sally wasn't on her case, not that Carrie was thinking about that. The thought with Carrie was just that, yeah, it sort of felt OK to be there, trying to make sense of it. Sally seemed to be more accepting, somehow, of what she was saying. Yes, just felt sort of easier somehow. It felt good. Just someone to talk to, someone who listened. She didn't want to be told what she couldn't do. And sometimes she did. She responded to Sally. 'They are but I can't keep drinking like this forever, can I?'

Sally shook her head. She had eye contact now with Carrie and she felt her heart going out to her. 'Wouldn't be very healthy.'

Carrie took a deep breath and sighed. 'But everything seems so horrible, and having a few drinks, getting pissed, really does make me feel good.'

'Mhmm. Yeah, and we all like to feel good, and drinking alcohol achieves that, quickly and reliably.'

Carrie listened. Although she wasn't thinking about it directly, she was hearing a greater softness in Sally's voice. It did feel easier sitting there, it was a word that kept coming back to her. She didn't think she'd ever just sat like this. What Sally had said was so true. She felt understood. It felt like she wasn't somehow alone with what she was trying to cope with, make sense of. Yes, she liked drinking, she felt good with it and yes, it was reliable – more than her parents were.

I have heard it said by clients when they have sought to make sense of why they turned to alcohol that part of it was that there was no one around to talk to. Sometimes it was more than just a part. A moment of desperation, a period where the future seems bleak, no sense of a way forward, maybe the result of a tragic loss or a build-up of problems that reaches a seemingly impossible degree, and alcohol eases things, takes one away from the anxieties, the stresses, the fears, the worries, the pain. And then it wears off. Still no-one to talk to, but the friend in a bottle is there, always available 24/7. You get the relief and the alcohol gets you. So it has been down the ages, and so it is today. And worryingly, more and more young people are bingeing, for many different reasons of course, but alcohol habits are getting established at an earlier age and society has to ask itself 'why?'.

Carrie continued to think. But she had her friends. She was seeing Maggs again regularly. She was different, her parents had really had a go at her about drinking and she was sort of reluctant to drink so much, and she'd said so as well. But Maggs didn't have the problems that she did. Her parents were always there for her. Maybe that was why Maggs seemed a good listener? Maggs hadn't criticised her for drinking, but had made it clear that she wanted to drink less. It seemed easier to hear it like that, and from a friend. As well as being grounded and having her parents discuss it with her – they hadn't gone into lecture mode – she'd also been quite shocked by what had happened. It had made her see alcohol differently and it didn't feel such an attraction to her.

Maggs' drinking isn't driven by the emotional and psychological need that Carrie experiences. She has a different relationship with it, because her drinking is less ingrained, and because she has fewer of her emotional needs invested in drinking and its effects, she is more able to step back and be open to an urge to change. It highlights how each person forms their own relationship with alcohol, each person ascribing their own meaning to the drinking experience. The counsellor will need to be sensitive to this. It is perhaps fortunate that Maggs is a friend of Carrie. Counsellors cannot do it all on their own. And where a young person is embedded within a family system that is not encouraging change, or is continuing to provide experiences that fuel the urge to drink, then friends, or maybe other relatives, can be the ones that offer the ongoing support and encouragement that the young person may need on a daily basis.

'I am drinking a bit less, it's like it just complicates things and, well, Maggs isn't really drinking much and, yeah, I like being with her.' She shook her head. 'But I still want to feel pissed.'

'Feel like getting pissed and drink to escape.'

'But I feel awful afterwards. It's not happening as much though. This last week I spent a bit more time with Maggs, she was with me when I broke my arm.'

Sally nodded.

'Well, she's changed, doesn't want to drink much. She's encouraging me not to, not going on at me, but sort of, I don't know, always suggests something else. She's good. She's a bit like you, she listens, you know?'

'Mhmm, she's really important to you and she's helping you. Sounds good.' Sally smiled.

'But sometimes I feel so confused by it all, by everything. I don't really know what I want. And, well, I hate what I'm feeling. It all builds up; only getting really pissed seems to make it sort of easier.'

Sally nodded again, acknowledging her agreement with what Carrie was saying.

'Only getting pissed gives you that relief, that ease.' Sally's thoughts strayed to her concerns as to what Carrie might turn to if the alcohol wasn't part of her coping mechanism, what she might turn to for that ease, to relieve the hurt, the emotional pain.

Carrie lapsed into silence and Sally's thoughts strayed for a moment to the number of young people – and not just young people – who self-harmed, who cut themselves to bring relief, or to give them a pain they could manage in contrast to that incessant emotional pain that could engulf you. Cutting localised the pain, externalised it, you could see it as well as feel it. You had control.

Carrie began to speak again. 'Messing around is OK, you know, having a laugh but it's not the same. I mean, yeah, we go to the cinema, that's a laugh, hang out in the town, but it's never the same, it's always still there.'

'None of that, what, goes deep enough?' Sally wasn't sure but felt she was capturing what Carrie was implying.

'I think of going home and I can feel it sort of creeping up on me from inside. It's horrible. It's like all of it is a distraction, takes me away from it a bit, yeah, sometimes it does, but it doesn't really take it away, not really.'

'And that's what you need, to take yourself away from what's inside you.' Sally felt that what Carrie had said really did sum it up. It doesn't take her away from what's inside her.

Carrie looked over to the window. It seemed to Sally that she was sort of looking for something in the distance, maybe looking for an answer, something out there to take her away. And yet Sally knew that it didn't work like that. Whatever you did, wherever you went, when you stopped you were still back with yourself again. For Carrie to change she needed to heal, and for that she needed to experience the human warmth, the attention, the love that it seemed had probably not been present in her life, or not present enough, or consistent enough. Yet she knew she had her friends, and Maggs was someone who seemed to be emerging as a significant person, and she had the counselling in which to experience unconditional positive regard and to begin to feel different about herself, if that was where her process took her – which Sally felt sure that it would, after all, it already was.

Sally found herself wondering whether Carrie had not felt love for a long while from her parents, or was it more recent? Her father sounded distant, remote, preoccupied. How long had her mother been drinking? Could the lack of love felt by Carrie have left her feeling unlovable, or even unloving? And how might she desperately seek that love? Currently she was using alcohol to blank out feelings; she knew how some young people – and not just young people – could turn to sex to get a feeling of being wanted, even to the point of putting up with abuse and exploitation, the closest thing they can experience to feeling loved. Yes, her heart went out to Carrie as she continued to sit there silently looking out of the window.

Sometimes, during a silence, a counsellor's thoughts may wander into speculation. What is important is that it is acknowledged and that they can bring their focus back to the client. There is a need to maintain therapeutic sensitivity towards the client as well as openness to one's own experiencing. It could be argued – and some who take a more energetic view of counselling might agree – that even though no words are being spoken and there is no eye contact, an energy interaction is continuing simply due to the fact that both people are in the room. Can a client experience the heartfelt nature of the counsellor's presence even though there is no eye contact or verbal responding?

If the notion that, in some mysterious way, energy does follow thought, that thoughts (and feelings) are not simply experiences locked inside the body of the experiencer, then how one thinks and feels towards one's clients during silences may well, at some subtle level, be making an impact or impression on the client, possibly at some organismic level rather than necessarily in awareness. If this hypothesis is correct, then it has application not only to the counselling session, but generally to how a counsellor thinks and feels towards their clients outside of therapy, and in particular the impact of the supervision session. What occurs in supervision may already be impacting on clients before their next meeting with the counsellor. Far-fetched? Maybe. But there is evidence as to the impact of thoughts and prayers on others in situations where there is no face-to-face or verbal contact. This is another intriguing area for further research specific to the counselling context.

The sense of searching was strong in Sally. She softly voiced it. 'Looking, searching for something?'

Carrie nodded, continuing to look out, her eyes moist with the tears that had begun to form. She didn't like to show her sadness. In fact her feelings tended more towards depression, but she knew she could feel sad as well. And now that sadness was what was most present. She felt a tear trickle over her eyelid and down her face. She sniffed. It dislodged another. 'How can I stop feeling like this?'

The question hung in the air. Sally felt momentarily uncertain how to respond. There was no answer, none that she could give, and it wasn't her role to give an answer anyway, and to just empathise with what had been said sounded false, somehow. As Carrie continued to look out of the window, Sally felt her heart going out to her. She felt close and yet sitting there she also felt sort of too far away. She moved her chair closer. 'How to feel different . . . how to feel different.' She spoke slowly, gently. There was nothing more to say.

Carrie nodded. It felt good that Sally had moved closer, she felt a little less alone with her sadness, and she seemed to just be there, be there with her, that was how it felt. And it felt good. She felt another set of tears running down her face. 'I want to feel different, Sally.'

Sally noted that this was the first time Carrie had called her by her name. She noted it and let it pass without comment. That wasn't the most important thing that Carrie was saying.

'Yes.' Sally paused. 'Yes, so? so want to feel different.'

Carrie took a deep breath and sighed. 'What am I going to do?'

Sally did not respond immediately, allowing Carrie's question to be present in both their hearts and minds. Carrie's words stayed with Sally. 'Do you know what you'd like to do?'

Carrie snorted slightly and shook her head. 'Get drunk, make myself forget.'

Sally took a deep breath, 'yeah'. She instinctively reached out and touched Carrie's arm reassuringly. 'Yeah. That's what you need to do.'

'Only way I know.'

'That makes me feel sad.'

'Sorry.'

'No need. I think it's only right that it should affect me that way.'

Carrie nodded slightly herself. Strangely she felt a kind of calmness amidst the sadness. She found herself shaking her head slightly as she sat tight-lipped, blinking. Another sigh, and then 'why don't they care about me?'.

'Feels like they just don't care?'

Carrie shook her head and pursed her lips. 'No, too busy with their own lives. I feel so tired, you know?' She felt herself start to yawn. 'I just feel as though I want to go to sleep.'

'Sleep yourself away from it all.'

Carrie heard Sally's words and could feel her presence. She was still holding her arm and that felt good. Her words were gentle, sort of floating her way, yes, just floating. Yet she also felt so alone inside herself as well. She wanted to feel held, the thought – it was more than a thought – but it was suddenly very present. She wanted to be held now, by Sally. She suddenly felt so small, as though the room had suddenly got bigger, the wall, the window seemed farther away, the ceiling felt higher somehow. She felt weird, spaced out, and although she wasn't thinking about it, she had begun to feel like a little girl. She turned to slowly face Sally who was herself experiencing spatial distortion in the room. Sally felt sure that Carrie was engaging with a deep part of herself, and she looked suddenly small, vulnerable, needy. She felt an instinct to hold her. 'You look like you need a hug.'

Carrie nodded. Sally reached over and held her. Carrie returned the hold. Feelings ripped through Carrie, feelings the like of which she had not felt before, deep feelings, powerful, sharp, intense. She felt weak, her breathing became shorter, she felt such a surge of emotion and burst into tears which became sobs as she clung to Sally. The emotion poured out of her. She'd never felt like this before and it felt as though it might go on forever. It was like a dam bursting inside of her. She felt utterly powerless to control it, she didn't try, she couldn't, she didn't want to, she was simply being the feelings, the emotions, that had engulfed her.

Sally continued to hold her, she had no choice. She closed her own eyes as she felt her own emotions rising to the surface as well. She sought to reassure Carrie who was continuing to sob between the almost otherworldly sounds of pain and distress. 'It's OK,' she spoke softly, 'let it out, let it go, it's OK.'

Carrie heard Sally, but her words seemed distant even though she was speaking so close to her ear, her own feelings were so intense, so present in contrast. She continued to sob; feelings not only of sadness but also feelings of being alone, of feeling so empty and yet feeling so full. So many feelings. She wasn't really thinking about them, they just were. She was being them, or they were being her. 'Oh dear, oh.' She swallowed.

'It's OK. Lots of feelings, all built up, had to come out.'

Carrie took a deep breath and began to ease her grip on Sally. She sniffed and let go, reaching for a tissue and then sat back in her seat to blow her nose. She dabbed at her cheeks and her eyes.

'A lot of emotion.'

Carrie swallowed again, she could feel the hot lump in her throat. She nodded. She couldn't really speak. Didn't feel like saying anything. Didn't know what to say anyway.

Sally sat quietly, keeping her attention on Carrie. She looked quite drained. Sally knew how the release of emotion could sometimes be energising, but sometimes leaves you feeling as if all your energies had been drained away.

Carrie dried her eyes, she was blinking and trying to regain her focus. 'Oh dear.' She blew out a long breath. 'I feel sort of lighter, tired, but sort of lighter.'

'Tired but lighter.' Sally smiled, seeking to reassure Carrie.

'My eyes are tired, but, I don't know, I-I don't know what happened. I just felt so, so, so ... ' Carrie swallowed and closed her eyes. The emotions remained so close, so present.

'Felt so ... ?'

'Small, alone. Lost. I-I sort of felt like I needed to be held.' Carrie hesitated, feeling anxious about what had happened, and a little embarrassed. 'Was that OK, I mean ... ?'

Sally nodded, 'Yes, yes I sensed it as well.'

'I don't get many hugs.'

'That's sad to hear.'

Carrie nodded. 'You get used to it. But, well, I mean, I do from friends, you know?'

'Mhmm.'

Carrie went quiet as a question formed in her mind. 'Is that why I drink?'

'Is that how it feels?'

'I think so. Sort of.' Carrie felt a little embarrassed still about what had happened and looked away, feeling herself flushing a little.

Sally noticed and decided to gently bring it into the open. She didn't want misunderstandings of the physical contact or anxieties to get established. 'You look a bit embarrassed, but it's OK, it happens, when we release deep feelings and emotions we can sometimes so need someone to hold on to, and someone to hold on to us.'

Carrie looked back, her momentary unease was passing. Sally spoke so caringly, and she was so right. That was what helped. She was so right, that was exactly what she knew she had needed, maybe still needed. She was aware of how the experience had left her feeling strangely lighter somehow. 'I do feel lighter, it's hard to explain, but it sort of feels like I've lost some weight, feel a bit less weighted down somehow.'

'Mhmm, less burdened maybe?'

Carrie nodded. 'It is why I drink, isn't it?'

'Very likely, it clearly seems to you to be linked.'

'If I could get rid of the feelings then maybe I wouldn't need to binge.'

'Maybe.'

The session was coming to an end. The recognition that Carrie had made for herself didn't need much more explanation. It was probably enough for Carrie to allow what she was now thinking and feeling to find its place within herself, within her self-perception. Sally checked that Carrie was feeling OK to head home and she said that she had a lot to think about. Sally suggested that she had had a very emotionally intense session, that the outside world might seem overwhelming, harsh, given the internal focus and sensitivity that she had experienced during that past hour. Carrie confirmed she would be aware of that and take things easy. They confirmed the date and time of the next appointment and Carrie left, still feeling lighter and aware that she was feeling a little disconnected with the world. Almost like after a few drinks, but not really the same. She sort of felt in control, more centred in herself. She felt clearer and yet the world around her felt strangely 'out there'. In a strange way while she liked to feel the effects of alcohol, the way she now felt seemed somehow more . . . , she couldn't really find the words for it. Like she was sort of more herself in some way. Maybe this is me, she thought to herself, a new me. She wasn't really sure what she meant by that but she knew she felt different, calmer, and wanted to preserve that calmness for a little while longer.

Points for discussion

- How did this session affect you? What feelings are you left with? How would you be dealing with these feelings if you had been the counsellor?
- How different do you feel Sally was in this session to the previous one?
- What were the key therapeutic moments in this session, and how did they arise? Consider this both in terms of the dialogue and person-centred theory.
- How appropriate was physical contact? What criteria would you use to decide?
- How did Sally convey her unconditional positive regard for Carrie?
- What do you feel Sally should take to supervision from this session, and why?

Write counselling notes for this session.

CHAPTER 12

Carrie attended four more sessions during which time she continued to talk of feeling lighter, although there were pockets of heaviness as well. But the trend seemed to be as if she was in some sense lightening her emotional load. She had more emotional releases, but none as intense as that one in the fourth session. She began to talk more openly about her drinking. It felt easier for her to do this now. It wasn't something she felt a need to deny or defend. She talked more about what she was drinking, and what it was like, although the amount and frequency had reduced. She described how having a few drinks made her feel what she described as 'normal', feeling how she needed, wanted to be. Carrie was able to differentiate the slightly drunk experience from the intense binge-ing-into-oblivion style of drinking and she was able to increasingly appreciate the roles each played in her life, in how she experienced herself.

Carrie still felt, and voiced, how unfair it seemed that she was having to think about what she drank, when others didn't care, but at other times she could see that she was right to do this, that it was what she needed to do. It was just difficult, sometimes, to feel different, feel sort of set apart. And then there would be times when she could see and acknowledge more strongly that she had to change for her own good, and that it was a positive choice.

She began to feel less intense at home. Although things didn't change a great deal, she did begin to talk more with her dad. He seemed to respond better to her, probably because she spoke more quietly, more reflectively in some ways, maybe more what some might describe as 'normally' in contrast to the 'everybody shouts' view that she had expressed in an earlier counselling session.

Maggs had also played a significant part, highlighting the importance of friends in helping and supporting people in making significant and difficult changes in their lives. Having a friend who had decided not to let her own drinking be such a central part in her life did make a difference.

The importance of peer pressure in contributing to young people drinking and using drugs receives a lot of emphasis, but there is also the peer pressure associated with not drinking and using drugs, with making different choices, and this is an important factor to consider and encourage. There have been a number of initiatives concerning drug and alcohol education involving young people, and they have generally been shown to have had a positive influence.

Carrie had also begun to express interest in the sessions about the effects of alcohol. She told Sally that it wasn't so much about herself, more for her mum. She felt she wanted to know more, understand how it affected people and why. Sally had told her about the health effects.

Conditions that can arise from heavy alcohol use include: liver disease including the development of hepatitis B and cirrhosis, stomach ulcers, oesophageal varices, heart disease and high blood pressure, cancers, pancreatitis, damage to nerves (peripheral neuropathy), diabetes, sexual and menstrual impairment, brain damage including alcohol dementia, Wernicke's encephalopathy and Korsakoff's psychosis. Mood is affected, mental health conditions can be exacerbated, suicidal frames of mind can develop. In short, alcohol is a toxic substance to the body, and wherever the blood goes, alcohol goes. And as well as the above, and perhaps more a factor for young people, there is the risk of alcohol poisoning, of accidents that are a direct result of being alcohol affected and of being the victim of another person's alcohol-fuelled violence.

Carrie's response had been that they don't talk much about that kind of thing at school, that most of the focus is on drugs. Carrie felt particularly interested in hepatitis B and the blood-borne viruses in general. She wasn't sure why they took her interest, but the thought that something could be passed on like that sort of made her feel quite uneasy. She felt that there should be more about that in schools. 'Maybe if they told us about these kinds of things first, made us aware of how we are at risk, you know, from picking things up from other people, and then told us how drugs and alcohol put us at risk.' Sally had agreed.

What seemed to be a significant change during the counselling sessions was the way that Carrie began to think more. She was less reactive, less driven by feelings, although she was aware of them. That also helped her to feel that 'lightness' that she had begun to experience.

She began to accept herself more, beginning to enjoy being herself. It perhaps helped that during this period the school term ended, but whereas in the past she might have used her free time to drink more, she and Maggs had decided to do things together without necessarily drinking, and if they did, not as much, though Carrie knew she found that difficult. It was like once she got a taste for it she didn't want to stop. She'd mentioned this to Sally in one session. They'd explored this difficulty. Sally empathised, and she also knew from what others had told her how difficult this could be. The alcohol hit the receptors in the brain and triggered feelings that drove a craving reaction. A drink wasn't enough. And then the desire, need, for the old, familiar experiences could take over. Sally felt sad that someone so young could already be having this reaction to alcohol. It was often present in people who were much older, with longer drinking careers, but already Carrie had developed her own chemical reaction to alcohol, fuelling an urge to drink more. What became clear was that Carrie had to learn to avoid alcohol, or somehow only drink when the circumstances put some boundary around how much.

Maggs and Carrie went to the cinema more, they'd go shopping, listen to music, all the usual things but it felt different to Carrie. It was as though she was beginning to be able to experience these things differently, be open to a different range of feelings and emotions to those that had begun to dominate her.

Carrie still didn't like school. She was glad term was over, but her attitude had softened. Rather than the hatred that she had expressed before, now it was more of a dislike. She felt more sadness than anger, particularly towards her mother, but in general for how her parents had become and how they were towards her. It wasn't so much that the sadness was new, more that she was more open to it. It had been present for her, but submerged under the hatred and buried by the alcohol. There was a kind of acceptance developing towards how they were, and an intention, a much stronger intention, to not let them get her down.

There were still periods when Carrie felt her mood dip, but they were not so frequent or intense. She was able to chat about them to Sally, chat being the word. It didn't drag her down the same. It helped to talk, as it stopped the internal pressure from building up as it did in the past. She realised that she could manage her feelings and not always be driven by them. It gave her a kind of a sense of that lightness, and she liked that.

The tone of the sessions was very different from the first three. More fluid, more openness. Carrie had grown to respect Sally more and more. And, yes, there were times when she wished Sally could have been her mother, or rather, that her mother could have been more like Sally. But she had to accept that her mother was as she was, hard as that was to accept, though she did still hope that she might change.

Sally had discussed at her next supervision session her sense that it was not just Carrie that needed therapy, but that the whole family system needed to be worked with. The pros and cons of a referral to a family therapy service were discussed. Sally felt sure that somehow the family system could be usefully addressed, that while Carrie was changing she was trying to change in what seemed a very unsupportive environment though, as she accepted, she had Maggs, and other friends seemed to be helpful, and her relationship with her father appeared to have improved. Following that exploration, Sally was left feeling that it could be helpful, though the question that remained unanswered was whether it would help Carrie's 'constructive personality change', or whether more difficulties might arise. How would her parents react? Would they both attend?

It was at the next counselling session that Sally mentioned to Carrie her discussion with her supervisor. 'I don't want this to sound like something you have to do, it isn't like that. But I was reflecting with my supervisor what else might help you, and we were thinking about your life at home, and how everyone relates to each other. And I wondered about family therapy.'

'Do you think it would help?'

'I honestly don't know, but I see you as having really changed a lot these past few weeks, and that your home life isn't really that supportive of you.'

Carrie had nodded. 'It's not easy. So what would happen?'

The idea of a referral to a family therapy service is not because it is believed that what is being offered in one-to-one therapy will not be enough, but so often a child's use of alcohol will be linked to processes within the family setting. Not every young person would agree to such a referral being made. It might need to be offered tentatively; however, with increasing concerns as to how parental substance use impacts negatively on children, there is a growing emphasis on the need to work with the whole family. Arguably more services of this nature should be established, specialist family therapy services working with substance-affected family systems. One such NHS service (only available to people from certain London boroughs) is listed at the back of this book.

Sally had explained about family therapy; in fact, there was a substance misuse family therapy service in the area, quite a unique service that specialised in working with families affected by a family member's substance use (including alcohol). Carrie had agreed. She'd also hoped that maybe it might help her mum as well. The referral was made. Sally was also mindful of the government's *Hidden Harm* agenda (Advisory Council on the Misuse of Drugs, 2003), raising awareness of the harm done to children and young people associated with parental drug (and alcohol) use.

The service agreed to take the referral and to initiate contact with Carrie's parents. They actually had a member of the team specialising in working with young people, and she would take the lead. They sought to be sensitive and to encourage the parents to understand that the referral was primarily to explore what would be helpful for Carrie. They would endeavour to be open and inviting, and avoid putting up barriers to the family's full involvement, though it was acknowledged this was not always easy, or successful.

The following counselling session takes place after the referral has been made, but before the family are seen.

Counselling session 9: more insights and reflections

Thursday 9 July

'Mum's anxious. She keeps asking me about why they need to come. Dad's OK, in fact I think he's a bit relieved, and we seem to be getting on better and better.

Yeah, he's still preoccupied with work; don't suppose that will ever change, but he makes time for me now and we talk about things a bit. I've told him a bit about coming here, how it's helping me. He seems genuinely interested. He also asks me about my day, what I've been doing and seems, you know, interested, though sometimes his mind is on other things. I point this out now and he usually agrees and it's usually work. Or mum. She's the problem.' Carrie paused. 'That sounds awful, but it's true. She seems to just drink and get depressed all the time. I don't know. Maybe something will happen. She needs to see someone, you know, someone like you. But she won't. She doesn't want to go to the family therapy appointment.' Carrie sighed. 'I don't think she will. I just have a feeling it will just be me and dad, but, well, that's OK. Maybe it'll be good for him too. He's agreed to take time off work. That's quite something, you know!' Carrie managed a smile. She felt that was quite an achievement.

'Something you seem really pleased about?'

Carrie nodded. 'I think deep down he needs to talk to someone as well.'

'Mhmm.' Sally nodded, not feeling there was more to say other than her acknowledgement of hearing what Carrie had just said.

'Can't be easy for him, you know, or any of us.'

'No, not easy at all.'

'But we get on better.'

'Mhmm, so you and your father, things are a lot better now.'

Carrie nodded. It felt like she wasn't so on her own now when she was at home, she felt as though – and it felt uncomfortable but true – she had a kind of ally, someone on her side, certainly in relation to coping with her mum, whose drinking remained such a feature of home life, but also generally. 'At least he's there for me a bit now. Not so on my own. I mean, I guess it helps not being at school as well. I can go out, do what I want to do, you know?'

'Mhmm, bit of freedom, chance to get away, do what you want to do.'

'Yeah, don't like being at home. Weather's been good too, that helps. Always get depressed when it's cold and wet. So it all sort of helps, you know?'

'Mhmm, sunshine, not being at school, your dad, it all helps.' Sally felt good about what she was hearing, while aware as well of a continued concern about Carrie's mother. Her drinking was clearly quite ingrained and she guessed it occurred most days, if not every day. She knew how it could dominate family life, the whole family system in a sense developing around the person who was drinking, either to support them or to scapegoat them. So often it went to one extreme or the other – eventually. Yes, there were so many factors that could contribute to mood change. Maybe counselling had come at the right time for Carrie; maybe she would use the summer to establish new interests and new sensitivities within herself, and perhaps strengthen further her relationship with her dad. Maybe she would try and reach out more to her mother, sometimes it happened, sometimes the child or young person would reject the parent. Either way, it could be quite extreme.

From outside it can be difficult to fully appreciate the pressures and tensions that can arise within an alcohol-affected family system. It is intense. It disrupts and distorts what might be considered 'normal' functioning. The impact on a child or young person can be that they gain what we might term a 'displaced sense of normal', and this can then become established within them as a normality to seek and relive. The chaos and uncertainty associated with the person who is drinking might leave them at risk of seeking a similar set of experiences – with or without alcohol. At an early age, a child may well internalise what they experience as being how it should be. It can become a foundational element within their sense of self. They might actually hate it, but still provoke it later in life. It can lead to huge psychological stresses as people keep repeating patterns that bring them distress and yet which they feel powerless to break free from. Often the original causes have to be addressed, the locked-up feelings from early times released, and the person given an opportunity to re-evaluate themselves within the experience of a therapeutic relationship, without the interference of negative and damaging conditioning influences.

Sally was also aware that Carrie's bonding with her father would probably isolate her mother more, and could lead her to drink more heavily. She could feel rejected, hopeless; so many powerful emotions could be present. She had no idea what fuelled Carrie's mother's drinking. She hoped she might make it to the substance misuse family therapy service and that this would be helpful and, at the very least, might help to improve intra-familial communication.

'It's strange, somehow I can sort of see how I got stuck, you know, like, yeah, like I wasn't going to hear anyone telling me what to do, or that I had a problem, or needed to change, all that stuff. I just wasn't there. Now it's feeling different.' Carrie paused. She tightened her lips. 'I'm feeling different, I guess.'

'You're feeling different.'

Carrie thought about what that meant to her. 'I feel sort of more positive, I don't know, it's hard to explain.'

'Sort of more positive, not easy to put into words, yeah?'

Carrie nodded. Gave her time to think, listening to Sally respond like that. 'I mean, I do get down days. Can't say why, just do. Wake up and know it. Feel different.' She shrugged and stuck her bottom lip out. 'It's how it is, I s'pose.'

'Mhmm, some days you just feel down for what seems no reason.'

Carrie nodded. 'Don't want to get up, just go back to sleep.'

'So, you wake up, know it's one of those days and just stay in bed.'

'Yeah. Usually days when I don't have anything planned much, like I don't know what to do, so I don't want to do anything.'

'Let me check I'm getting this right. It's on days when you don't have anything planned when your mood, what, sometimes lowers or always lowers?'

'Sometimes.' Carrie paused, thinking about it a bit more. 'Yes, definitely not always. But when I have things planned it's OK. Yeah, things can irritate me but I've got things to do, things I want to do.'

'Something about having things you want to do . . .'

Carrie nodded.

'And that's important, and maybe something different?' Sally smiled as she responded. Yes, she thought, something to want to do rather than just doing things to feel better or not feel at all.

Carrie was nodding now. It was. She wasn't sure what else to say and lapsed into silence, turning slightly to look out of the window.

Sally sat and watched Carrie, aware of thinking to herself how much Carrie had changed, in some ways she was almost unrecognisable as the young girl who had come to counselling those two months or so back. 'Carrie, I know that you're having your own thoughts at the moment, but I'd like to say how much I'm aware of how much you have changed, how much more positive you seem to be, more open, less closed, less defensive.'

To Carrie that felt good and seemed to catch something of what she was feeling in herself. It hadn't been exactly what she'd been thinking, her thoughts had been simply about the things she looked forward to. Yes, she knew it wasn't all perfect, she wasn't sure it ever would be, but she hoped that it might. 'I do feel more positive, and I guess that now when I feel down I sort of cope with it. It's like I sort of know it will pass.'

'Mhmm, like you relate differently to it, knowing it will pass?'

Yes, thought Carrie, I do feel positive. She felt herself smile. There was mum. She felt a lot of concern, maybe more concern in a way. Now that she didn't feel so angry all the time, she sort of felt worried, wanted to help, do something.

Sally noticed the sigh and responded, 'but still things to sigh about.'

Carrie nodded. 'I hope mum gets help. She doesn't want to, well, just takes anything said about her drinking as criticism. Hmm.' Carrie paused. An uncomfortable realisation had come into her thoughts. 'Hmm.' She remained silent a little longer, feeling she ought to say what she was thinking, but also not wanting to. Like she didn't want to hear herself say it, and yet felt that she had to as well. 'Bit like I've been.' Another pause. 'Hadn't thought of it like that.' Another pause as words came to mind. She spoke them. 'We all need someone to talk to, don't we?'

'You mean everyone, or everyone in your family.'

'Both, I guess, both.' Carrie had actually been thinking about her family. Sally's response has sort of affected her focus in some way Left her hesitant for a little while. It took her time to regain her focus.

A difficult moment. The counsellor was unsure and sought to clarify, but in so doing disturbed the client's focus. A response that simply highlighted the family might have been better. Had it been wrong, the client could have corrected the counsellor. But had it been right then the focus would have been held, unaffected by a distraction emerging from the counsellor's frame of reference. Perhaps the counsellor was being a little too clever. Or maybe there was some other thought in her mind that provoked her sense of uncertainty as to what the client was referring to.

The session continued with Carrie talking about school and not being sure what she wanted to do when she left. She again said how much she didn't like school. Sally responded by highlighting how Carrie had been experiencing a phase of life in which she had seemed to hate so many things.

'I don't know if I can feel different about school. It seems a bit distant at the moment, anyway, being summer. I can't imagine feeling different.'

The tone of the counselling interaction had changed. It seemed as though it was two people chatting about something. Sally noticed it but decided to stay with it.

'You didn't think you could feel different towards home.'

'Yeah, but it's been about escaping. I guess I have less to escape from now. Things are sort of easier at home, sort of, but not really as well. I guess I sort of feel easier about things, maybe, I don't know. Maybe if I keep seeing you it'll get different. I don't know, can't imagine feeling different about school.'

'Hard to imagine feeling different about school.'

Carrie nodded.

A question had formed in Sally's mind. Was it helpful to ask it? It was emerging from her frame of reference, quite clearly, and yet it felt very present, and it felt as though she must decide in the moment, to think about it too long would simply take her focus away from Carrie. It felt as though the dialogue between them had become sort of different, it felt like it didn't have the same deep, therapeutic undertone. She voiced her question. 'A question has just come into my mind, I'm wondering what has made you feel different.'

'Being listened to.' The response was immediate and without hesitation. 'Took a while to get used to it. Guess I was so used to not being listened to, being always told what to do. Didn't like it when you did that to me, though.'

'What, tell you what to do?' Sally winced, thinking back to those early sessions and how she had clearly come across to Carrie.

'Yeah, but I've changed. This is now my escape, isn't it?'

Sally recalled that Carrie had mentioned escaping a little while back and she hadn't responded, hadn't shown empathy, hadn't shown she had heard it. She sensed its importance.

'Coming here replacing how you used to escape?'

'Sort of. But this lasts longer. Sounds strange that. But it does. You get pissed, fall asleep, next day, well, shit again, you know?'

Sally nodded.

'But this lasts longer. I feel calmer and that's strange and good as well. I don't sort of react to things the same; don't get pissy with people, you know?'

'Mhmm.' The session continued in a similar reflective style. It felt like a bit of a process of taking stock of the journey so far. Unplanned, unforced, but it had

emerged. The conversation shifted to shopping. It was Carrie who had introduced it. She wanted to know which shops Sally liked. Sally decided to be open
in her responses. The tone became increasingly conversational. Sally accepted
that for whatever reason this was what Carrie wanted, perhaps a kind of conversation that she might not have often had with an older adult. She warmly
accepted that it was how Carrie wanted and needed to be, and actually quite
enjoyed the conversation.

There are times when what might be termed 'conversational counselling'
emerges within sessions. While some might consider this inappropriate, my
view is that it largely depends on what is happening in the therapeutic
relationship. Such 'conversation' can have therapeutic value. It can allow
other aspects of the client to emerge and come into relationship with the
counsellor in a way that more traditional counselling responses might
not allow for. For the person-centred counsellor it must emerge from the
client, and must feel 'right' within the therapeutic context. In this instance,
the client may be avoiding feelings by being conversational, but equally
she may be experiencing a new way of being that is bringing a particularly
satisfying experience. To have such a conversation, to know that one can
have such a conversation and get good feelings from it offers a therapeutic
process and experience for the client. The process is trusted. The client is
warmly accepted. Her need to express herself is appreciated. For me, this
is therapeutic.

The session came to an end. The next session would be the first after the family
therapy appointment. Carrie mentioned it again, and said she was feeling
anxious, but determined to go through with it. Sally wondered if the conversational tone had been Carrie's way of coping with it, preferring to talk about
something she felt good and comfortable about, rather than something she
was anxious about. Well, it was a better way of handling discomfort than
drinking. And Sally felt no need or urge to point that out. She trusted Carrie's
own process. It was her experience, she had been able to be how she needed to
be. She did just wonder whether the 'feel-good factor' from shopping might in
time become a replacement for the drinking. But then, well, it was naturally
human to choose to do things to make ourselves feel better. It was when the
choice was made continuously to the point that there was no control that it
could become such a problem.
After the session Sally reflected on the sessions so far. So many different experiences, so many different features to the journey. It did seem that Carrie was
becoming more self-aware, more able to choose how she wanted to be, rather
than being simply driven to reaction by feelings and emotions that over-
whelmed her. She had said how important being listened to had been. Being
listened to. What did people really mean by that? She felt she wanted to check
that out with Carrie. Maybe next time, or some other time. Was it actually

being listened to, the attention, when she was speaking? Or was it hearing the counsellor respond verbally, letting the client know what they have heard or experienced in response to what has been said? To feel listened to? To feel heard? To be listened to? To be heard? Empathy so often seemed such an important factor in the relational experience for clients. So many people have their inner worlds locked up inside them, hidden away, so much psychological energy invested in maintaining concealment – not just from others, sometimes from themselves as well. And carrying that around. She shook her head.

So many young people can carry secrets about their families, or their own secret fears. Or secret pain that they have felt unable to share, coming out as sadness or anger, or a host of other emotions. And then there was alcohol, the quick fix in a bottle or a can. Make you feel different – fast. Make you forget – temporarily. Make you loosen up – but too much and you might lose your step, fall over. So many young people, Sally thought, encountering alcohol at an earlier and earlier age, bingeing themselves into another world. Some would come out undamaged, others not. Some would resist the temptation to continue bingeing, others not. Some would end up with a lasting relationship – with alcohol.

Points for discussion

- How has this session left you feeling? How has the counselling process with Carrie affected you? Has anything changed in you as a result of participating in her process?
- What were the significant features of the counselling process so far, and which seemed most therapeutically helpful, or unhelpful, and why?
- What are your thoughts and feelings towards the dynamics of the relationship between Carrie and Sally? How would you describe it in the language of person-centred theory?
- What do you imagine the family therapy session will be like?
- What are your hopes and concerns regarding the likely impact of this on Carrie?
- What would you take to supervision from this session, why, and what would you hope to gain from it?

Write notes for this session.

An alternative scenario for Carrie

It is perhaps worth reflecting on how life might have turned out for Carrie had she not had her alcohol use responded to at the accident and emergency department, and had she not had counselling or any intervention to help her resolve her problems and bring her alcohol use under control and make different lifestyle choices. The following could have been the summary of Carrie's life a few years on . . . It may seem extreme, but it happens the world over, and is happening to young girls as you read this.

It was a few days after the incident. After a short stay in hospital, Carrie had returned home. Nothing much had changed. Her mum was still drinking heavily, her father working and he had been drinking a bit more as well with Carrie being away, and they were still rowing. They both got their act together when they visited Carrie, with neither of them wanting anyone to know about how they felt about each other.

Carrie's arm had healed and her experience had shaken her, but it wasn't long before she was continuing to drink again. And that's how it was for the next few years. She left school with little in the way of qualifications and was pregnant at 16. She'd been to her GP a number of times following the accident, but apart from a few general comments about her need to watch her drinking, very little was actually said.

Carrie miscarried, but her drinking continued, in fact it increased. She was now very much chemically affected and was also using other substances as well, particularly cannabis, but also amphetamine and ecstasy. She liked the energy, the boost, the feeling different, the range of experiences – up and down, so long as it was intense. Her drug and alcohol use continued to escalate and she began to work in the sex industry, at first picking up clients herself, but later she got into a relationship with a guy who took her on and pimped for her. He was abusive, only interested in the money he could get for her. Carrie was treated badly, subjected to physical and sexual abuse, and raped on a number of occasions. He introduced her to heroin, said it would make her feel less tense all the time.

She continued to sell her body – she had no choice. She was in fear for her life if she tried to break free. She had tried to get away on one occasion, but had been brought back and beaten savagely. She drank and used drugs – supplied to her by her pimp, and she was now dependent on him to meet her need for drugs.

There was no glamour in her work – she wasn't working for a higher class escort agency. This was the gutter end of the sex industry and she was trapped, hating herself, her parents, everyone who was making her do the things she had to do to be sure of that next fix. By now she was heroin dependent but also drinking heavily as well. She was HIV positive from unprotected sex and, as she jacked up the heroin with her shared needle, she was quite unaware that the hepatitis C virus was already making its way into her bloodstream to add to the hepatitis B that was already attacking her liver. There were no thoughts about this, no concerns, she simply did what she had to do, to try and feel a little better.

Reflections

Carrie reflects

I never thought about my drinking being a problem, well, you don't, do you? Everyone drinks. Wherever you go, there's alcohol. And the government is telling us you can drink, what, 24/7? Places staying open later and later. So what's the problem? Seems they want us to drink more, and then they tell us not to. Doesn't make much sense to me.

I think I'll always, you know, want a few drinks. Maybe not like I did. But I don't want to never get off my face. I mean, that's what people do. I don't want to be any different. Don't get me wrong, my attitude's changed. I feel better for not drinking like I did, but I won't be one of those people that never drinks.

Yeah, I didn't want counselling, didn't see any point. I was wrong, I can see that now. Felt like I was sort of picked on, so many of my mates drink a lot as well. I suppose I should be grateful. And I am, sort of. I guess, well, yeah, things might have been difficult if I'd carried on like I did. I guess I am grateful, just still feel I might be missing out on something. I guess, well, yeah, guess I've learned that you've got to treat alcohol with a bit of respect and be aware that it can have a bad effect. But you just don't really hear that enough, my friends don't think like that, everything sort of tells you drinking's the cool thing to do, you know?

The counselling has been good, having someone to talk to. Didn't like it to begin with but, yeah, it has been good. Wish things would change at home, though. Can't seem to get mum to accept she's got a problem. I suppose I can sort of understand that now, but I really wish she'd accept help. She didn't come to the first family therapy appointment, dad and I went. It was good. They were really nice. I just wish mum would come. They said they'd see her on her own if she preferred. They just want to try and help her feel able to come along. They told us not to push mum too much, be gentle, emphasise how it will help us all to be like a family. I'd like that. Can't remember when it was like that, not really.

I suppose I think about her more now. Before, well, I was either getting pissed, or getting over being pissed, and just being a pain I suppose, particularly at school. Now I worry about her. And I know I can't make her change, they told us that, but I just wish I could . . . I mustn't ever be like mum.

Makes me wonder how many more parents will be like mum in the future with so many young people binge drinking. I can see how it'll be a big problem. Can't make sense of why they make alcohol more available. Just seems to be asking for trouble if you ask me . . . not that anyone does. Who, really, seriously, asks us young people what we think?

182

Author's epilogue

You have travelled part of a journey through the lives of Gary and Carrie. Each had their own reasons for binge drinking, and each, gradually and in their own way, realised for themselves a need to change. In both cases, their alcohol use was linked to relational experiences in their lives, centred on their family situations.

Not all young people will, of course, binge drink for the reasons illustrated here. The reasons are many. Some will be dealing with issues by their drinking, or it may be driven by conditioning factors from their experience of life. Others will binge drink simply because it is what is available and what others are doing – Maggs is an example of this. Her emotional investment in alcohol was significantly less than Carrie's, and her parents took time and trouble to talk it through with her, while being firm and consistent in their response in grounding her. She realised her need to be different. It was less of a struggle for her to release herself from her developing relationship with alcohol.

Gary had his own reasons for drinking and his own struggle with his alcohol-fuelled behaviours. He was unaware of why he was drinking, not appreciating that his behaviour was more extreme than others', and certainly not seeing it as a problem. He just thought he was out for a laugh and a pull with his mates, unaware that other forces were at work within his nature.

For Carrie, alcohol offered release from the feelings she had towards herself and her life. An escape, a way to feel better, different. Whether pissed or heading for oblivion, alcohol satisfied her need. She could so easily have died, asphyxiated in her own vomit, before she could have even made it to counselling and given herself a chance of something different. Life can be like that, death and life can hang on an experience, a choice, an outcome to a single event.

Change, of course, is not always easy, and not always quick. The processes in this book may be viewed as being somewhat compressed. Yes, young people change at their own pace, everyone does. It is my view that sustainable change cannot be hurried and must be genuinely owned by the person themselves as something they not only need to do (a mindful process) but also want to do (a heartfelt response). The two play their part, and arguably both need to be present. Perhaps there is research potential here to see how these two distinct motivations affect the process of change.

Person-centred counselling offers the opportunity for young people to experience a positive, self-affirming and constructive relational climate. This may be new to them and require some adjustment. Or it may be something that they have experienced in their lives before. Either way, it provides for the possibility of constructive personality change – indeed in thinking about children and young people perhaps we should think more in terms of constructive personality development. This, it seems to me, is an important aspect of what the person-centred approach offers and which again could be a focus for more research. As highlighted in the Introduction, Rogers and others have written about the application of the approach within the educational environment.

So, Gary and Carrie will move on into their respective futures, avoiding the alternative scenarios offered for them both had they not received or responded to interventions in relation to their alcohol use. Of course, it is speculation, but my hope is that what you have read will ring true. So many young people are seriously harmed by binge drinking, and some of the harms have yet to arise for the young binge drinkers of today.

Finally, there are Rick and Sally, both working to form therapeutic relationships with young people who struggle to accept that they have problems. It's not an easy area to work in. Both took their processes to supervision, seeking to ensure they could be more effectively and authentically present to continue their therapeutic work with their clients. We should not underestimate the importance of supervision, perhaps more so when working with young people. I say this because the relational dynamics can become very complex. The urge to help, to minimise harm to the young person can obstruct the relationship-building process in some instances.

My hope is that, having read this latest volume in the *Living Therapy* series, you will feel a greater sense of empathy towards young binge drinkers, and feel yourself able to be authentically and sensitively present with them, whatever stage they may be at, in terms either of their drinking or of their perception of their drinking along the problematic continuum. Society does not offer much to help young people cope with alcohol. It is advertised everywhere, glorified at times in the media, and generally treated with disrespect. With young people establishing entrenched drinking habits at earlier ages, we must expect to see the serious harms to health emerging at earlier ages.

Our society shows increasing signs of alcohol dependence. And, like a problem drinker, it is finding it increasingly difficult to acknowledge that it has a problem, a serious problem. 'I can handle it', 'it's just a phase', 'it has more benefits than harms'. We hear individuals say this about their own binge drinking. But when a society is being harmed by alcohol, yet continues to say that it can handle it, that it's just a phase, that the benefits outweigh the harms, then there are serious questions to be asked. The phenomenon of young binge drinkers is a sign and a symptom. Something is wrong. But let's not rush into simply blaming them. We would do well to seek to understand what it is, in our society, that makes alcohol such an attraction and, it seems, such a necessary prerequisite to feeling good for so many of today's young people.

References

Advisory Council on the Misuse of Drugs (2003) *Hidden Harm: responding to the needs of children of problem drug users.* Home Office, London. www.drugs.gov.uk/ReportsandPublications/National Strategy/1054733801/hidden.harm.pdf

BBC News (2005) http://news.bbc.co.uk/1/hi/uk/4134772.stm (accessed 19 October 2005).

Beich A, Thorsen T and Rollnick S (2003) Screening in brief intervention trials targeting excessive drinkers in general practice: systematic review and meta-analysis. *British Medical Journal* **327**: 536–42.

Bentall RP (1990) The syndromes and symptoms of psychosis. In: RR Bentall (ed.) *Reconstructing Schizophrenia.* Routledge, London,

Bien TH, Miller WR and Tonigan JS (1993) Brief interventions for alcohol problems: a review. *Addiction* **88**: 315–36.

Bozarth J (1998) *Person-Centred Therapy: a revolutionary paradigm.* PCCS Books, Ross-on-Wye.

Bozarth J (2002) Empirically supported treatments: epitome of the specificity myth. In: JC Watson, RN Goldman and MS Warner (eds). *Client-centred and Experiential Psychotherapy in the 21st Century: advances in theory, research and practice.* PCCS Books, Ross-on-Wye, pp. 168–81.

Bozarth J and Wilkins P (eds) (2001) *Rogers' Therapeutic Conditions: evolution, theory and practice. Volume 3, Unconditional positive regard.* PCCS Books, Ross-on-Wye.

Bryant-Jefferies, R (2000) An exploration on the theme of congruence, incongruence and alcohol use. In: D Bower (ed.) *The Person-Centered Approach: applications for living.* Writers Club Press, Lincoln, USA, pp. 233–55.

Bryant-Jefferies R (2001) *Counselling the Person Beyond the Alcohol Problem.* Jessica Kingsley Publishers, London.

Bryant-Jefferies R (2003) *Time Limited Therapy in Primary Care: a person-centred dialogue.* Radcliffe Medical Press, Oxford.

Cooper M (2004) Towards a relationally-orientated approach to therapy: empirical support and analysis. *British Journal of Guidance and Counselling* **42**: 4

Embleton Tudor L, Keemar K, Tudor K, Valentine J and Worrall M (2004) *The Person-Centered Approach: a contemporary introduction.* Palgrave Macmillan, Basingstoke.

Evans R (1975) *Carl Rogers: the man and his ideas.* Dutton and Co, New York.

Everall RD and Paulson BL (2002) The Therapeutic Alliance: adolescent perspectives. *Counselling and Psychotherapy Research* **2**(2): 78–87.

Gaylin N (2001) *Family, Self and Psychotherapy: a person-centred perspective.* PCCS Books, Ross-on-Wye.

Hallam RS (1983) Agoraphobia: deconstructing a clinical syndrome. *Bulletin of the British Psychological Society* **36**: 337–40.

Hallam RS (1989) Classification and research into panic. In: R Baker and M McFadyen (eds) *Panic Disorder.* Wiley, Chichester.

Hallet R (1990) *Melancholia and Depression. A brief history and analysis of contemporary confusions*. Masters thesis, University of East London.

Harris B and Pattison S (2004) *Research on Counselling Children and Young People: a systematic scoping review. British Association for Counselling and Psychotherapy, Rugby.*

Haugh S and Merry T (eds) (2001) *Rogers' Therapeutic Conditions: evolution, theory and practice. Volume 2, Empathy.* PCCS Books, Ross-on-Wye.

Health Development Agency (2004) *Binge Drinking in the UK and on the Continent.* Health Development Agency, London.

Jenkins P (2002) *Young People's Rights to Confidential Therapy in the Healthcare Setting. Healthcare Counselling and Psychotherapy Review. Vol 2.* British Association for Counselling and Psychotherapy, Rugby.

Joseph S and Worsley R (2005) *Person-Centred Psychopatholoy: a positive psychology of mental health.* PCCS Books, Ross-on-Wye.

Kirschenbaum H (2005) The current status of Carl Rogers and the person-centered approach. *Psychotherapy* **42**: 37–51.

Kutchins H and Kirk S (1997) *Making us Crazy: DSM: the psychiatric bible and the creation of mental disorders.* The Free Press/Simon Schuster, New York.

Levitt BE (2005) *Embracing Non-directivity: reassessing person-centred theory and practice for the 21st century.* PCCS Books, Ross-on-Wye.

Mearns D and Cooper M (2005) *Working at Relational Depth in Counselling and Psychotherapy.* Sage, London.

Mearns D and Thorne B (1988) *Person-Centred Counselling in Action.* Sage, London.

Mearns D and Thorne B (1999) *Person-Centred Counselling in Action* (2e). Sage, London.

Mearns D and Thorne B (2000) *Person-Centred Therapy Today.* Sage Publications, London.

Merry T (2001) Congruence and the supervision of client-centred therapists. In: G Wyatt (ed.) *Rogers' Therapeutic Conditions: evolution, theory and practice. Volume 1, Congruence.* PCCS Books, Ross-on-Wye, pp. 174–83.

Merry T (2002) *Learning and Being in Person-centred Counselling* (2e). PCCS Books, Ross-on-Wye.

Miller WR and Rollnick S (1991) *Motivational Interviewing: preparing people to change addictive behavior.* Guilford Press, New York.

Norcross JC (2002a) Empirically supported therapy relationships. In: JC Norcross (ed.) *Psychotherapy Relationships that Work: therapist contributions and responsiveness to patients.* Oxford University Press, Oxford, pp. 3–16.

Norcross JC (2002b) Empirically supported therapy relationships. In: JC Norcross (ed.) *Psychotherapy Relationships that Work: therapist contributions and responsiveness to patients.* Oxford University Press, Oxford.

Orford J and Velleman R (1995) Childhood and adult influences on the adjustment of young adults with and without parents with drinking problems. *Addiction Research* **3**: 1–15.

Patterson CH (2000) *Understanding Psychotherapy: fifty years of client-centred theory and practice.* PCCS Books: Ross-on-Wye.

Poikolainen K (1999) Effectiveness of brief interventions to reduce alcohol intake in primary health care populations: a meta-analysis. *Preventative Medicine* **28**: 503–9.

Rogers CR (1939) *The Clinical Treatment of the Problem Child.* Houghton and Mifflin, Boston.

Rogers CR (1942) *Counselling and Psychotherapy: newer concepts in practice.* Houghton Mifflin, Boston.

Rogers CR (1946) Significant aspects of client-centered therapy. *American Journal of Psychology* **1**: 415–22.

Rogers CR (1951) *Client Centred Therapy.* Constable, London.

Rogers CR (1957a) The necessary and sufficient conditions of therapeutic personality change. *Journal of Consulting Psychology* **21**: 95–103.

Rogers CR (1957b) Personal thoughts on teaching and learning. *Merrill-Palmer Quarterly* **3**: 241–3. Wayne State University Press. Reprinted in: H Kirschenbaum and VL Henderson (eds) (1990) *The Carl Rogers Reader*. Constable, London, pp. 301–4.

Rogers CR (1959) A theory of therapy, personality and interpersonal relationships as developed in the client-centred framework. In: S Koch (ed.) *Psychology: a study of a science. Vol. 3: Formulations of the person and the social context*. McGraw-Hill, New York, pp. 185–246.

Rogers CR (1967a) *On Becoming a Person*. Constable, London (originally published in 1961).

Rogers CR (1967b) The interpersonal relationship in the facilitation of learning. In: R Leeper (ed.) *Humanizing Education*. NEA, Washington, DC, pp. 1–8. Reprinted in: H Kirschenbaum and VL Henderson (eds) (1990) *The Carl Rogers Reader*. Constable, London, pp. 304–22.

Rogers CR (1969) *Freedom to Learn: a view of what education might become*. Charles E Merrill Publishing Co, Columbus, Ohio.

Rogers CR (1977) The politics of education. *Journal of Humanistic Education* **1**: 6–22. Reprinted in: H Kirschenbaum and VL Henderson (eds) (1990) *The Carl Rogers Reader*. Constable, London, pp. 323–34.

Rogers CR (1980) *A Way of Being*. Houghton-Mifflin Company, Boston, MA.

Rogers CR (1986) A client-centered/person-centered approach to therapy. In: I Kutash and A Wolfe (eds) *Psychotherapists' Casebook*. Jossey Bass, California, pp. 236–57.

Slade PD and Cooper R (1979) Some difficulties with the term 'schizophrenia': an alternative model. *British Journal of Social and Clinical Psychology* **18**: 309–17.

Steering Committee (2002) Empirically supported therapy relationships: conclusions and recommendations on the Division 29 task force. In: JC Norcross (ed.) *Psychotherapy Relationships that Work: therapist contributions and responsiveness to patients*. Oxford University Press, Oxford, pp. 441–3.

Strategy Unit (2003) *Interim Analytical Report*. Cabinet Office, London.

Strategy Unit (2004) *Alcohol Harm Reduction Strategy for England*. Cabinet Office, London.

Tudor K and Worrall M (2004) *Freedom to Practise: person-centred approaches to supervision*. PCCS Books, Ross-on-Wye.

UK Government (2003) *Interim Analytical Report*. HMSO, London.

UK Government (2004) *Alcohol Harm Reduction Strategy for England*. HMSO, London.

UK Government (2005) *Youth Matters* (Green Paper). HMSO, London.

Velleman R (1993) *Alcohol and the Family*. Institute of Alcohol Studies, London.

Velleman R (1995) Resilient and un-resilient transitions to adulthood: the children of problem drinking parents. In: *Alcohol Problems in the Family*. IAS Conference Report. Institute of Alcohol Studies, London.

Vincent S (2005) *Being Empathic*. Radcliffe Publishing, Oxford.

Warner MS (1991) Fragile process. In: L Fusek (ed.) *New Directions in Client-centered Therapy: practice with difficult client populations*. Chicago Counseling and Psychotherapy Center, Chicago, Monograph 1, pp. 41–58.

Warner MS (1997) Does empathy cure? A theoretical consideration of empathy, processing and personal narrative. In: AC Bohart and LS Greenberg (eds) *Empathy Reconsidered: new directions in psychotherapy*. American Psychological Association, Washington, DC, pp. 125–40.

Warner MS (2000) Person-centred therapy at the difficult edge: a developmentally based model of fragile and dissociated process. In: D Mearns and B Thorne (eds) *Person-Centred Therapy Today*. Sage Publications, London, pp. 144–71.

Warner MS (2001) Empathy, relational depth and difficult client process. In: S Haugh and T Merry (eds) *Rogers' Therapeutic Conditions: evolution, theory and practice. Volume 2, Empathy*. PCCS Books, Ross-on-Wye, pp. 181–91.

Warner MS (2002) Psychological contact, meaningful process and human nature. In: G Wyatt and P Sanders (eds) *Rogers' Therapeutic Conditions: evolution, theory and practice, Volume 4, Contact and perception*. PCCS Books, Ross-on-Wye, pp. 76–95.

Weiner M (1989) Psychopathology reconsidered. Depression interpreted as psychosocial interactions. *Clinical Psychology Review* 9: 295–321.

Wilk AI, Jensen MN and Havighurst TC (1997) Meta-analysis of randomized control trials addressing brief interventions in heavy alcohol drinkers. *Archives of Internal Medicine* 12: 274–83.

Wilkins P (2003) *Person Centred Therapy in Focus*. Sage, London.

Wyatt G (ed.) (2001) *Rogers' Therapeutic Conditions: evolution, theory and practice. Volume 1, Congruence*. PCCS Books, Ross-on-Wye.

Wyatt G and Sanders P (eds) (2002) *Rogers' Therapeutic Conditions: evolution, theory and practice. Volume 4, Contact and perception*. PCCS Books, Ross-on-Wye.

Useful contacts

Person-centred

Association for the Development of the Person-Centered Approach (ADPCA)
Email: adpca-web@signs.portents.com
Website: www.adpca.org

An international association, with members in 27 countries, for those interested in the development of client-centred therapy and the person-centred approach.

British Association for the Person-Centred Approach (BAPCA)
Bm-BAPCA
London WC1N 3XX
UK
Tel: +44 (0)1989 770948
Email: info@bapca.org.uk
Website: www.bapca.org.uk

A national association promoting the person-centred approach. It publishes a regular newsletter *Person-to-Person* and promotes awareness of person-centred events and issues in the UK.

Person Centred Therapy Scotland
Tel: +44 (0)870 7650871
Email: info@pctscotland.co.uk
Website: www.pctscotland.co.uk

An association of person-centred therapists in Scotland which offers training and networking opportunities to members, with the aim of fostering high standards of professional practice.

World Association for Person-Centered and Experiential Psychotherapy and Counselling
Email: secretariat@pce-world.org
Website: www.pce-world.org

The association aims to provide a worldwide forum for those professionals in science and practice who are committed to, and embody in their work, the theoretical principles of the person-centred approach first postulated by Carl Rogers. The Association publishes *Person Centred and Experiential Therapies*, an international journal which 'creates a dialogue among different parts of the person-centred/experiential therapy tradition, supporting, informing and challenging academics and practitioners with the aim of the development of these approaches in a broad professional, scientific and political context'.

Alcohol use and young people

Addaction Central Office
67–69 Cowcross Street
London EC1M 6PU
UK
Tel: +44 (0)20 7251 5860
Fax: +44 (0)20 7251 5890
Email: info@addaction.org.uk
Website: www.addaction.org.uk

Addaction is a leading UK charity working solely in the field of drug and alcohol treatment. Founded in 1967, it now has over 70 services across the UK from Glasgow to Penzance. Addaction also offers services in some areas specifically for young people.

Adfam
Waterbridge House
32–36 Loman Street
London SE1 0EH
UK
Tel: +44 (0)20 7928 8898
Fax: +44 (0) 20 7928 8923
Email: admin@adfam.org.uk
Website: www.adfam.org.uk

Adfam is a community committed to ending the silence about drugs and alcohol, and placing the needs of the family at the heart of society's response. It supports families by providing literature, training programmes, online information and direct support; informing families by listening to their needs, and producing relevant information from their feedback; challenging policy makers and social stigma by highlighting the real impact substance use has on families in the UK.

Alcohol Concern
Waterbridge House
32–36 Loman Street
London SE1 0EE
UK
Tel: +44 (0)20 7928 7377
Fax: +44 (0)20 7928 4644
Email: info@alcoholconcern.org.uk
Website: www.alcoholconcern.org.uk
Telephone information line Monday to Friday, 1.00 pm to 5.00 pm on: +44 (0)20 7922 8667

Alcohol Concern produces a comprehensive series of factsheets which include *Young People's Drinking*.

Alcohol Focus Scotland
2nd Floor
166 Buchanan Street
Glasgow G1 2LW
Scotland
UK
Tel: +44 (0)141 572 6700
Fax: +44 (0)141 333 1606
Email: enquiries@alcohol-focus-scotland.org.uk
Website: www.alcohol-focus-scotland.org.uk

Alcohol Focus Scotland (formerly the Scottish Council on Alcohol) is a national voluntary organisation for alcohol issues, and is committed to improving the quality of people's lives by changing Scotland's drinking culture – promoting responsible drinking behaviour and discouraging drinking to excess.

Alcoholics Anonymous
General Service Office
PO Box 1
Stonebow House
Stonebow
York YO1 7NJ
UK
Tel: +44 (0)1904 644026
National Helpline: +44 (0)845 769 7555
Website: www.alcoholics-anonymous.org.uk

Connexions Service
Connexions is for young people aged 13–19 years, living in England and wanting advice on getting to where they want to be in life. It also provides support for young people up to the age of 25 who have learning difficulties or disabilities (or both). This modern public service involves young people in its design and delivery.

The service is managed locally by 47 Connexions Partnerships around the country that bring together all the key youth support services.

Connexions Direct is part of the Connexions Service, offering information on a wide range of topics as well as confidential advice and practical help. Connexions Direct advisers are there to listen without judging and are available to talk to from 8 am to 2 am, 7 days a week, and can also give callers details of their local Connexions Partnership.

Tel: +44 (0)80 800 13219
Website: www.connexions-direct.com

All calls to Connexions Direct are free from a landline and an adviser will ring back to your mobile. The Connections Direct website offers a facility for young people to email in questions as well.

Drinkline
Tel: +44 (0)800 917 8282

A national drink helpline providing information, support and advice for drinkers of all ages. Callers can be put in touch with local specialist services. Calls are free and do not appear on your bill (except for mobile phones).

The Institute of Alcohol Studies
Alliance House
12 Caxton Street
London SW1H 0QS
UK
Tel: +44 (0)20 7222 4001
Fax: +44 (0)20 7799 2510
Email: sales@ias.org.uk
Website: www.ias.org.uk

Substance Misuse Family Therapy Service
Unit 5
1–31 Elkstone Road
London W10 5NT
UK
Tel: +44 (0)20 8960 0880

The Substance Misuse Family Therapy Service is a specialist psychotherapy service offering individual family-focused sessions, couple marital therapy, and whole-family sessions for anyone affected by drink or drug use, including non-users. Although the referral service is only available to a limited number of London boroughs, the Substance Misuse Family Therapy Service can respond more widely to general enquiries related to drug- or alcohol-related familial problems.

Index